IF YOU WOULD JUST

Get Out of Bed

My Life with
Chronic Fatigue Syndrome

BY STEPHANIE KELLEY

If You Would Just Get Out Of Bed

Published by: *KK Bell, LLC.*
202 N. Curry St. #100
Carson City, NV 89703

Printed in the United States of America
ISBN # 0-9742710-0-4
This publication is designed to tell the author's story and is
for entertainment purposes only. It should not be used for
medical advice, diagnosis, or treatment. If you or someone you
know suffers from any symptom described in this work, it
is important to seek professional medical assistance.

Names have been changed to protect identities.

Table of Contents

ACKNOWLEDGEMENT

*W*hen I first decided to write this book, I wasn't sure if I would have enough material to compile into a manuscript. But a strange phenomenon took place. The moment I sat down at the computer and started typing, I couldn't control the amount of information I wanted to share. Page after page began to take shape and I found myself struggling to maintain some order to my thoughts and feelings.

I could finally discuss how I felt without anyone interrupting me — no one told me how I *should* feel or what I *should* think. I was able to be honest and sincere for the first time.

I truly felt the full range of emotion throughout this process. At times, I laughed. Sometimes, I was mad. But the most intense feeling was pain. I cried as I wrote the words. I believe that is why it is so honest. I never planned to have anyone read it. The book was strictly for me — a form of catharsis, I guess.

A great number of people have participated in creating my story. Some more negative than others, yet all integral in the person I have become. And oddly enough, I appreciate and thank each and every one of them.

Now I struggle to find just the right words and hope I don't leave anyone out.

Mike - you have been my strength and my best friend — I will forever love you. Mom and Dad - thanks for believing me when so many others didn't. I hope I will always make you proud. Pete and Silje — I will always appreciate your kind souls. You've helped make one aspect of my life much easier. Jeff and Firuzeh — thanks for all the love and compassion. It will never be taken for granted. Zachy — I love you, and I want you to know and feel compassion. I hope this will be one way for you to learn it someday. Moorea — you've always quieted my soul with your kind and gentle spirit. I love you! And all those who were unkind, you've strengthened my character and I'm learning to forgive.

Thank you Gisela at Picante Creative for the amazing cover. You truly captured the hope and peace I wanted to portray. It was a pleasure working with you.

Finally, a huge thanks to A-1 Editing Service for all their input and their kind compassionate manner. Ed and Patti — you turned a mass of words into a story, and Nicole — you made a terrifying process so much easier.

Thank You!

Prologue

*A*s I stood in the back of the church on my father's arm, waiting to walk down the aisle, I could not help but be overcome by the emotion of the moment.

In a few short moments, I was going to become Mike's wife.

My father looked at me, and for the first time in my life I saw tears in his eyes.

"I'm so proud of you, and all you have done. I love you so much." He struggled to stay composed.

I hugged him. "I love you too. Thank you for everything... my whole life."

At that moment, the "Bridal March" began, and with my parents on either side of me, I took my first steps toward my new life.

Few guests in the church could appreciate the impact of this simple walk down the aisle, and even fewer understood the tremendous fight I had waged to get to this amazing day.

"In sickness and health..." had never had as much impact as when Mike said those precious words to me.

After years of defeat, I finally had a victory. For it was not long ago that I was not able to get out of bed.

Now — a new start, a new husband, a new name.

The beginning of a life blessed with peace and love — not pain and hopelessness.

Mike vowed to stand by my side — and I his. I now know that I will never be alone.

I cannot imagine the feelings my parents were experiencing. Pure joy to finally see their daughter shine and find true happiness, and utter sadness over the idea of "giving her away". They stood by my side through so much agony, and now it was time to step back and allow someone else to step into their coveted role.

I have suffered from Chronic Fatigue and Immune Dysfunction Syndrome (CFIDS), also known as Chronic Fatigue Syndrome (CFS), for years. In fact, I can trace it back to when I was about twelve years old.

Doctors have tried for years to explain, in excruciating detail, why the disease exists, but have not yet been successful. One theory has it as a virus; another would blame it on bacteria, and even a third, a yeast infection.

Regardless, the fact remains that millions of people suffer debilitating fatigue everyday, without a diagnosis and with no treatment in sight. CFIDS is a disease of complete and all-consuming exhaustion. Along with extreme fatigue, a myriad of other symptoms includes migraines, cognitive disorders, appetite changes, sleep pattern disruptions, swollen lymph nodes, sore throats, memory loss, and muscle and joint pain...

These are just a few of the dozens of symptoms CFIDS patients suffer from daily. The degree and severity varies from individual to individual, but many victims find the disease dramatically interferes with their everyday life. It affects their ability to work, play, and care for themselves.

Many sufferers sleep eighteen to twenty hours a day and find the simplest of daily tasks all but impossible. Taking a shower, brushing their teeth, cooking a meal, working a normal job, and even talking on the phone become monumental tasks CFIDS patients find insurmountable.

The symptoms are vague and many other diseases are suspected before CFIDS is considered. However, extreme fatigue and the inability to access normal amounts of energy remains the common thread throughout all patients.

CFIDS is defined by the following:

1) Patient must exhibit severe fatigue lasting six or more months that cannot be explained by any other medical condition.

2) During the severe fatigue, the patient must exhibit at least four of the following symptoms:

- impaired short-term memory and concentration
- sore throat
- tender lymph nodes
- muscle pain
- multi-joint pain without swelling or redness
- headaches of new type, severity, pattern
- unrefreshing sleep
- post-exertion malaise lasting more than 24 hours

Unfortunately, at this time, there is no treatment. There is no magic pill to stop or reverse the effects. Once patients become sick, they have to wait it out. For some, like me, it can be months at a time. For others, it can be years.

At some point during their illness, patients seek medical attention — only to find doctors are unsympathetic. Many medical professionals believe the symptoms are imagined — and most doctors do not validate how they feel. Unbelievably, victims hear doctors' claim CFIDS doesn't exist.

For years, the medical community has betrayed the victims of this disease, and led them down a path of self-doubt. Some start to believe they are lazy, depressed, and worthless.

After all, they have been raised to trust and believe the medical community. Doctors swear an oath to help those in medical need, but many times, they are the first ones to turn their backs on CFIDS patients. Why can't a doctor admit there might be something out there they don't understand — something beyond their grasp? Instead, they run test after test and tell patients they are perfectly healthy.

Throughout the history of medicine, doctors have been faced with new and challenging diseases. Cancer was once thought to be highly contagious and people alienated its victims. HIV and AIDS were so misunderstood that the general public was afraid to have any contact with sufferers. Victims are still stereotyped — no matter what the transmission route. Unfortunately, the list goes on and on.

With CFIDS, doctors and scientists have yet to find any cause, test, cure, or treatment. It has been lumped into the "unknown" category. Therefore, some dismiss it all together. Others, link it to diseases such as fibromyalgia (a disease of unexplained joint and muscle pain that overlaps the symptoms of CFIDS), lupus, multiple sclerosis, rheumatoid arthritis, and even AIDS.

So CFIDS patients continue to hope for some sort of help.

Many doctors encourage victims to exercise and push themselves harder. However, when the patient takes their advice, they become sicker then ever. It is a vicious cycle that adds to their feelings of doubt and shame.

To add insult to injury, there is no test for CFIDS. There is no way for the medical community to confirm the existence of the disease. Even worse, doctors who do believe the victims, have no treatment in their arsenal to help.

Finally, the families and friends of the CFIDS patient start to raise an eyebrow at their illness. "You look fine," they say, and they start to doubt.

They ask questions, and make remarks like:

"She's so lazy!"

"I'm sick of hearing her complain!"

"Why does she always cancel plans at the last minute?"

The ones closest to the CFIDS patients often scream in frustration and back out of their lives. As a result, the victims quickly lose faith in their trusted friends and beloved family members.

Patients often find themselves trying to justify, in some small way, how they feel. The medical community has abused them, the general public has abandoned them, but they always expect their loved ones to be their support and guiding light. Sadly, those who love them can sometimes be the cruelest.

CFIDS starts slowly by creeping into your life. It silently robs you of the things you find most dear. If you could recognize it, you might be able to fight it, to wage some sort of defense strategy against it. Unfortunately it doesn't make its presence known until it is too late.

In fact, the diagnosis is given when nothing else can be found — it is used as a "catch-all". Every blood test returns normal and the doctor has exhausted every diagnostic tool at his disposal — he does not know what else to tell you. The news can be devastating, and the sheer terror of a "diagnosis" unimaginable.

Unfortunately, this is my story.

I have experienced the most callous thoughts and deeds, and been overwhelmed by kind words and gestures. I know the pain of ridicule, and the joy of a little compassion. I have experienced the agony of losing friends and a career I loved because of CFIDS and clung for dear life to my family — who always stood by my side.

I know how it feels to have a doctor laugh in my face, and the elation of finding one who is able to shed a tear at my suffering. Unfortunately, I am all too familiar with self-doubt, fear, pain, and anger.

Worst of all, I know the terror at the prospect of a life altered by severe fatigue and the thought I might never again leave my bed.

However, through it all, I have been able to strengthen my character and have learned to embrace the disease that has permanently changed my life.

After my diagnosis, I started to scour the Internet. I read every piece of material I could find. I soon learned this disease was mocked, laughed at and not taken seriously.

I do not think I could have fathomed the amount of adversity I would face over the following years. There were books about crazy diets, insane exercise rituals, and scary alternative medicine options. However, there was no information on what it is really like to live with it every day.

In addition to my own problems, I had a wonderful family who did not have any idea what to do. How could they cope? What about their emotional roller coaster ride? How could they help? There was no material to guide them either.

The only useful information I saw was on a talk show in the mid-Eighties, ten years before my diagnosis. A woman explained what it was like to have a disease called Chronic Fatigue Syndrome. I remember listening to her story thinking what a wretched life she must lead, and secretly realizing how I could relate to her struggle.

At fifteen I recall knowing, in some strange way, watching this woman explain how hard it was to get out of bed, that this was going to be my story.

Over the years I have cried out for information that might let me know I am not alone. Doctors laughed at me, my family cried over their sick daughter and sister, friends got sick of hearing I was not feeling well — and the public continued to think I was lazy.

Now I am hoping to help patients, doctors, families, friends, and the community. I want victims to know the disease is real — and the pain they feel is legitimate.

I want people to understand the destruction CFIDS can wreak on a precious life. I hope, in some very small way, I can validate those who feel lost — and let them know the light at the end of the tunnel shines brightly.

I was humiliated and embarrassed to admit how much I suffered every day. I allowed this disease to consume my life for many years — and it defined who I was. Everything I claimed to be revolved around this syndrome.

I struggled so long for help, and I knew — despite the criticism — I was sick. I would sit in the exam room crying and begging the doctor to help me, only to hear that I was perfectly healthy and they could find nothing wrong.

After my diagnosis, I thought I could finally start to make sense of what was happening to me — and explain why I was always so sick. However, the more I learned about CFIDS, the more doubt I felt, the more questions I had, and the less answers I found.

I hope my story can help sufferers know that they are not alone, and give loved ones, caregivers, doctors, and the public a small glimpse into the unquestionable suffering surrounding a disease many in the medical community say doesn't exist.

Most people who are sick with Chronic Fatigue Syndrome are too ill to speak for themselves, but I am fortunate enough to have healthy, vibrant times — and it is important for me to speak for all of those who cannot.

It is time to make all people aware!

It is my time to take a stand!

If You Would Just Get Out of Bed

I was living an active and reasonably normal life in my early- and mid-twenties, but I could never escape the underlying exhaustion that was always present. I always burned the candle at both ends. From holding down multiple jobs, to working twelve- to fourteen-hour shifts, something had to give.

Before I realized it, small changes were starting to take place. They crept up so silently I almost did not notice. I would make plans with friends on Monday to go out on Friday, but when Friday would come around, I would fight with myself all day about whether or not I wanted to go.

I would spend the day at work thinking, "Should I go? Okay, I'll go but just for a few hours."

Then, just as quickly, "No I don't think I'm going to go."

Using an excuse was always good. I thought friends would understand if I had some sort of symptom that would impair my ability to have a good time.

So I would think, "Is that a headache coming on? Well, if I have a headache then I definitely shouldn't go."

Then I would think about how much fun I would have if I went — and I wanted to go so badly.

"No, wait — this is stupid," I reasoned, "I'm going to go."
My internal struggle would rage all day, but the end result was always the same. I would cancel at the very last minute and it did not take long for my friends to stop calling. They grew tired of hearing my creative excuses.

Next, I would find that I started to plan my sleep. If I went to school in the morning, and had to work in the evening, I would calculate exactly how much sleep I could get in between. I would practically run out of the classroom to my car and race home because it might mean I would get an extra fifteen minutes of precious sleep.

If class went long, I would subject myself to excruciating mental anguish. My entire day would be ruined if I had to stop and get gas, and I had not calculated that into my sleep time. I knew, when I would lie down I needed to sleep for at least two hours or I would wake up feeling far worse than before I went to sleep. Most of the time, my naps would last for four hours or more. And when I did wake up, I was groggy and nauseous. It would take time for my head to clear, and I would hurt all over.

I also used this ritual at night. I would lie in bed and calculate how many hours I could get before I was due to wake the next morning. In fact, I probably lost a tremendous amount of sleep worrying about it. In the morning, I would look forward to the sleep I would get later in the day. I would promise my body, *Just four more hours until I can lie down.*

I started to plan my entire life around sleep. Appointments and commitments were scheduled with the idea that I had to be able to sleep. I never scheduled something in the morning and then something else in the evening; there was too much of a time gap. If I did, it was guaranteed that one, the other, or both would be cancelled.

I knew I was stronger in the late afternoons and early evenings, so I tried not to plan anything in the mornings or mid-afternoons. I found excuses not to be available early in the day. I even changed my work schedule to the swing shift so I would be able to get the excessive amounts of sleep I was beginning to require.

I realized that during the night I needed at least twelve hours of precious sleep. During the day, I needed three to four, and at my sickest, I slept about eighteen hours a day.

The next thing CFIDS stole was my desire to maintain my personal hygiene. I would start to put off showering. Even when I did shower, I avoided washing my hair as long as possible. Just the idea of holding up my arms to scrub my head was exhausting. At one point, I cut my very long hair so I would not have to work so hard to wash, condition, and brush out my locks.

Soon, I had to start sitting down in the tub to bathe myself because I could not stand and cleanse without getting so dizzy I would almost pass out. I was afraid to shower without someone in the house. I feared blacking out, and hurting myself. My mom offered to help with my showers and my hair, but I think that was, for me, the ultimate humiliation. I was starting to become weaker; my motivation was waning, and my passion for life fading.

Brushing my teeth was a huge chore. My parents finally bought me an electric toothbrush because I was unable to brush my teeth the old-fashioned way. I would have to sit down and rest after just a few manual strokes of a toothbrush.

Our ability to care for ourselves is a luxury we often take for granted. Imagine having trouble getting out of bed to go to the bathroom. Imagine putting it off as long as you can because you can barely lift your arms off the bed.

I would have to urinate so badly, but I just could not muster the strength to get up to use the restroom.

From there, CFIDS struck the final blow. I started to realize I was becoming unable to work. The job that I loved, the very way I defined myself. CFIDS stole it out from under me. I was unable to care for animals anymore. My whole purpose in life — my absolute passion.

At this point in the progression of the illness, I was able to look back and see how much I had actually lost. It crept up on me so silently I had barely noticed before. The magnitude of loss and change was staggering. I could not believe the amount of pain I was experiencing.

Within a few days, I needed to take a leave at my job. Indefinite really, because I did not know how long this bout would last. I would guess four to six months based on the past, but there was really no way to know. I was fortunate I had supportive parents who always believed I was sick, and who allowed me to live at home through all of this.

At this point, I had to start filling out disability forms and fight the government. After all, I paid money into the system, and darn it I deserved it!

I filled out the appropriate forms after receiving them in the mail. I made sure my doctor signed them, and I put them in the mail myself. Now the waiting game began. If I did not work at all, I had a much easier time receiving my benefits. It was set up on an automatic payment system that spit out a check every week.

However, when I worked a few hours a week and had to report those hours to the disability office — all hell broke loose.

I would fax and mail the appropriate, government-supplied paperwork every week detailing the exact hours I worked. Every week, the fax and mailed copy were not received.

When I had not received a check for a couple of weeks, I called and talked to one of the infamous government employee operators. She said my benefits had been cancelled because I had not responded to whether or not I worked during a particular week.

Infuriated, I asked what needed to be done to reinstate my benefits and she explained that I could fax the hours I worked to the disability office. I agreed and inquired about whom I should call to verify that the fax arrived.

"No one, you have to wait ten days until it gets in the system," she quipped.

"Well then, do you have a direct line that I can call you back on if there is a problem?"

"No ma'am, there are nine centers throughout the state that take these calls."

"So I won't be able to reach you if I call back?" I am seething at this point.

"Only if you happen to get this call center. Have a great day!"

This continued for about four months. I would follow-up on my faxes and they would, of course, claim they never received them. All the while, I had no money. Finally, an operator who sensed I was at my breaking point took all the hours I worked for the last four months over the phone and authorized a check to be sent to me the next day.

But the cycle started all over again. I faithfully submitted my paperwork, and the disability office faithfully lost it.

Why should I have to fight so hard? I was trying to get better, and I would waste my time trying to solve this ridiculous problem. What a tremendous amount of stress they were inflicting on people.

I was now entering my sick time. My daily routine was usually the same. I slept about twelve hours during the night. When I got up in the morning, I ate a little something and within an hour or two, I would be back in bed. I would wake about four hours later and, depending on the time might have some lunch or dinner.

Sometimes I would talk to my parents for a little while, but usually I would lay on the couch and watch TV. Most days, I would take a second nap; this one would only be two to three hours. Again I would get up and watch a little TV and then go to sleep for the evening. It was easy for me to sleep up to twenty hours a day.

Friends stopped calling altogether by this time. Work stopped checking in to see how I was. But my parents were always there. I am sure they felt I would be better off if I got out of bed and moved around. But they watched how sick I would get with small amounts of exertion.

There would be mornings when they would want to go to breakfast and then have errands to run. They were so wonderful, they would let me pick the place to eat, and then bring me home and drop me off before they would go out.

I would get so tired I felt like I was going to vomit if I did not lie down right that second. Many times I would have to lie down in the back seat of the car. I could not sit up long enough to get home. I never thought I could desperately need sleep.

One night we had tickets for the theater. When we talked about it a few weeks before, it sounded like a lot of fun. We went to dinner before the show and half way through the meal, I became so weak and pale that we finished quickly and my parents took me home. There was never a bad word said to me about the cost of the ticket or the inconvenience I had caused them. I would bet they were late to the play that night.

My parents showed me nothing but compassion, and I think it has had a lot to do with why I have been able to cope with all of this. Through it all, they have tried to stay upbeat and happy, and have always encouraged me to do the same.

I lived at home until I was twenty-eight years old (other than a year here and there) but they never complained. In fact, when they were ready to retire and move to a new home, they always looked for a house that could accommodate me, should I need their help.

So many times, people would tell me I slept too much.

Doctors would tell me to get out of bed and exercise. They assured me I would feel better. I tried all of these little tidbits of advice, and would force myself to get up and walk, but the repercussions would last for days.

I would try to stay awake, but I felt as if I had the flu and was unable to do even basic tasks. I had no option but to sleep. My body was in a constant state of extreme exhaustion.

This pattern has repeated itself every year for the last five or six years, and I find myself in bed for months at a time. Over the years, I have found little things I believed have helped, and I would always think I found my cure; my silver bullet. I figured it was over, CFIDS was no longer a part of my life, and I would not have to deal with it anymore.

But before I knew it, that same exhaustion would creep back into my life. Once again, I was wasting my life away in bed.

Can You Understand My Frustration?

My toughest battle was always with myself. I took pride in being a hard and dedicated worker. I was never unmotivated or lazy. In fact, as much as I hate to admit it, I am a very type-A personality. I am compulsive and obsess over just about everything I do. From working out, to work, to dieting, to writing this book. I do everything as though my life depended on it.

When I decided to start working out, all the books I read on CFIDS said to start with one or two five minute walks a day, but I would do twenty minutes of power walking. Then, within a few days, I would be running.

After working a ten-hour shift, I frequently stayed another four hours because, in my mind, the hospital could not run without me. After all, who could do the job better than I?

When I decided to lose weight and start a diet, I had one cookie in four months and felt guilty that I allowed myself the forbidden pleasure.

And when I decided to write this book, I could not sit down for ten minutes here and fifteen minutes there. I would write for hours at a time.

I am always SO driven. I feel that if I am going to do something, I must be the best, the fastest, and the most versed. I cannot just be mediocre. My competitive spirit rears its ugly head almost all the time. On the outside, I do not think people can see all of this turmoil going on. It is an internal struggle that goes on constantly in my mind. At work, at home, in relationships. Could this never-ending personal fight contribute to my declining health?

I have tried to understand why my body decides, one day, that it is time to shut down. Why it feels so abused it cannot continue. Before I know it, my body has stopped. But, unfortunately, my mind keeps fighting. The internal struggle becomes slightly different, yet tremendously harder.

After my body fails, I start making bargains with myself. If only I can get through a shower, I will sleep for the rest of the day. My mind makes deals with my body. I ask it to just hold out a little longer and I will reward it with precious sleep. I offer myself sleep now in exchange for being able to go to the store later. But my body always wins out. The trip to the store always waits until tomorrow. And tomorrow always turns into the day after.

Eventually, I become so exhausted that I am unable to cook or prepare food. I try to figure out ways to make eating as simple as possible. Something canned or boxed. If it has more than two or three steps, or I have to watch it on the stove, it won't happen. As a result, my diet begins to decline. I start eating less because I can only get up to eat once, maybe twice, a day. And I start to binge because I get so hungry.

I am now in bed for most of the day, and I soon start to get mad at myself for my sheer laziness.

I'm a healthy young woman! I scream at myself.

I push myself to get up and get moving — but the repercussions last for days. Before I know it, my body wins and against my will, my mind gives up. I cannot keep up the impossible fight against such a strong opponent. I stop arguing with myself, and start to accept what is becoming my new reality.

Unfortunately, this devastating defeat now causes me to become unable to process multiple thoughts. I start to get confused easily and things I found simple before have become very difficult.

Just watching television is too much to bear. I stare blankly at the screen, and try to understand the story line unfolding in front of me. Simple shows I used to enjoy become hard to focus on. My attention span has dramatically shortened, and a half an hour show feels like an eternity. I am barely able to follow the plot of a simple commercial.

Television was the one thing that helped pass the time, but I find sleep works better.

If I have a boyfriend, he gets mad and frustrated and wants some sign from me that I care. He cannot and does not understand that I am fighting everyday to conserve my energy so I can go to the bathroom without having to stop and take a nap afterward. I am fighting for my life and his need for validation is very low on my list of concerns.

I can barely meet the very basic needs of my own life, and he is complaining because I am not meeting his.

I get so annoyed at people who keep telling me I need to learn how to make them feel special when I am in the middle of the hardest fight of my life.

I am sick of being told I need to be chipper and in good spirits all the time. Don't they understand I want nothing more than to laugh — instead of cry?

I feel so hurt by people who say that they MUST have CFIDS because they took a nap last week, and have been tired today. I would trade my soul to feel that way. It is so condescending.

I get so angry with people who say they knew someone with CFIDS and all they had to do was stand on their head and close one eye and now they are fine. Is it impossible for them to understand if it was that simple, I would have been cured years ago?

And I get so frustrated with people who try to fix it for me. How hard is it to sit back, listen, and let me cry on their shoulder? I will ask for help when I need it.

I have learned not to talk to everyone I meet about CFIDS. People do not really care. When they ask you how you are, they do not really want to know. Most people at my various jobs have been aware I have health problems, but they do not know what I have, or to what extent I suffer.

Most of the time, I put in twelve- to fourteen-hour days. Suddenly, within a day, I am gone. Most people say they had no idea anything was wrong with me. That is exactly how I want it. I do not want to be treated differently, nor have people feel sorry for me. I do not want people to ask me how I am all the time. Most of all, I do not want people to think I am lazy or faking my symptoms. I do not want them to talk behind my back, and question the validity of my suffering. In fact, I am still embarrassed to say I even have it.

I had a co-worker at a job many years ago who claimed she suffered from fibromyalgia. At first, I tried to be sympathetic, because after all, I can understand how hard it is to have people not believe you. However, after a while, I started to doubt the legitimacy of her illness.

I worked in the cubicle next to her and I found that every day, she was informing everyone about how terrible her life was because of this disease, and how she never felt well. She would sit on the phone for hours with family and friends and relive, in excruciating detail, every ache and pain. Throughout each and every day, at least ten people would stop and ask if she was feeling better. She would grimace and cringe whenever someone was looking directly at her. At times, she would hunch over holding her stomach, and cry out in pain.

But when no one was watching, or she was pre-occupied with the little bit of work she did do, the pain seemed to not exist.

She had an uncanny way of mimicking symptoms from various people in the office. I suffered from migraines, and within a few months, coincidentally, so did she. I had ovarian cysts, and after my trip to the emergency room one evening for a rupture, she seemed to develop terrible ovary pain. It got so bad that I was afraid to say anything at all because I did not want to hear her infamous, "I have that too!"

It did not take very long for people to start to wonder if her complaints were real or whether she used it as an attention-getting mechanism. The dramatic behavior never existed when she thought no one was watching.

She wanted everyone to think she was such a martyr. In reality, she was out running a few miles every day, was working forty to sixty hours a week, had a reasonably active social life, and was only "sick" when it was convenient — and only when it would get attention.

I often wondered if she acted this way at home and what her family and friends thought of the behavior. In the meantime, I was struggling to put in my few hours a week at work and was strapped to my bed, sleeping most of my life away. The ironic part was no one had any idea I was suffering as much as I was.

As exhausted as I was, I never felt the need to doze off while people were looking in my direction; I did not need people to acknowledge my illness every time I saw them.

Those who are really sick and suffer through these terrible diseases do not want the world to know. We are usually laughed at, people do not believe us, and the last thing we want is to be put in a situation where we might be ridiculed.

The medical community has already shunned most of us, and our pain runs deep from that betrayal. The very people who take an oath to help us turn around and tell us we are making our symptoms up, suffering from depression, and are lazy.

I always believed if I were diagnosed with a "legitimate disease", people would rally to support me. They would wear colored ribbons, hold parades, send in money, collect information, and proudly proclaim that they support me. They would say how strong I was and what a brave soul I am in the face of tragedy. They would talk to everyone they knew about alternative treatments, and would understand why I was retreating, and did not call so often. They would respect me when I said I did not feel well, and would not be mad at me because I could not meet them for lunch.

But the diagnosis of CFIDS manifests itself differently in those who claim to love its victims. Instead of the support and friendship, people start to gossip with each other. They start to wonder if you are for real (just like I did with my co-worker).

There are no parades and no colored ribbons dedicated to the cause. Extremely small amounts of money are being donated, and that which is gets misallocated to other research. Most people quickly forget their so-called friends and loved ones, and move on with their lives.

There is no understanding when a victim cannot go to lunch. They tell themselves this is the last time they are going to ask. There are no telethons, no campaigns, no commercials, no talk shows, no information. So we continue to feel totally alone.

Support groups are hard to find because we cannot, and will not, commit to a certain day and time. After all, the participants do not know if they will be able to even come to a meeting — let alone participate in one.

For some strange reason, people have a much easier time explaining and understanding a "legitimate disease". They can put their finger on what it means.

They can see a tumor on an x-ray or MRI, they can see the needle marks from the blood work, and they can see the incisions from surgeries.

With CFIDS, there is nothing to put your arms around. There are no cold hard facts, no scars, or obvious markings. There are no masses or deformities. We usually look "totally healthy" — but we are living a death every day.

Put yourself in a CFIDS victim's shoes for a moment. Try to sleep eighteen hours every day for four months. Imagine being so weak you crawl to the toilet and struggle to get onto the seat. Try to fathom climbing the stairs in your home, only to be so tired at the top you have to lie on the floor and rest before you can catch your breath. Stop and think how it feels to know you need help bathing yourself because you cannot do it on your own. And, just for a moment, try to imagine living through this, and knowing no one believes you.

These are just small pieces of the tremendous fight people with CFIDS wage every day.

I do not want to diminish the suffering experienced by victims with "legitimate diseases", but I feel ripped off. This has been my life for more than fifteen years, and still, I am humiliated by it. I've been embarrassed to tell people how much I suffer.

I should be able to stand up, admit I have CFIDS, and know people will support me. I should feel confident that I will not be ridiculed.

CFIDS is one of the loneliest and scariest diseases for its victims. Not only does it "not exist", but there is no treatment, and no cure. It affects every aspect of my life and can strike a powerful blow at any time. It can rip apart my spirit, and shred my dignity with not so much as a hint of regret. It steals from me the things I value the most, and it does not even bat an eye.

After each bout, in addition to putting my body through rehabilitation, I have to work hard to rebuild friendships, and put my life back together. But just when I start to feel comfortable and like life is back on track, CFIDS strikes even harder.

All of my progress gone.

All of my personal accomplishments have been destroyed.

The hope it will not happen again is shattered.

I get my hopes up and CFIDS continues to kick me in the face — over and over again. Every day, I wonder if today is the day. Will I be able to get out of bed? Will I be in bed for the next six months? I feel like a time bomb waiting to go off.

And usually, for those of us who suffer, it is a matter of time.

First Recollection

I started having health problems when I was quite young. My first recollection was when I was about 12 years old.

I was out playing baseball in the street with the local kids in the neighborhood and I started to have stomach cramps. I went home early, which I never did, and my mom thought I might be constipated.

She was having a meeting that night, so I went upstairs into our loft and watched TV. My mom came up to check on me a few times through the evening and the pain seemed to get progressively worse. What was slight discomfort had developed into strong gas cramps. I went to bed early that night, hoping to wake up in the morning free of the pain.

At one o'clock that morning, I woke in agony. I went to my parent's room. They decided to take me to the emergency room because the pain had become so severe. On the way down to the car, I ran to the bathroom and threw up.

We arrived at the ER and the first thing they did was administer an enema. At 12, I was horrified and humiliated. In fact, I think after all was said and done, the emergency room doctor gave me three enemas.

This, unfortunately, did not change the pain and the doctor decided to admit me to the hospital overnight for observation. My parents were scared to death to leave me by myself, but the nurse told them to go home and get some rest. I was right next to the nurses' station and they would keep a close eye on me. So, reluctantly, they left.

My parents called me the second they arrived home and my mom was hurt when I told her that it was nice to be alone. She told me recently how scared she was when they left — they had never felt so helpless. That was my first night alone — ever!

The next day, the doctor ordered a consultation from a gynecologist. After the exam, they decided I had a ruptured ovarian cyst. It was an assumption really, because I was so young and I do not remember an ultrasound being done.

A year or two later I went to Lake Tahoe with my family. We spent the days skiing and the evenings with my aunt and uncle in their cabin. On the way home, I broke with my first cold sore. It was on the tip of my nose, of all places, and swelled to an unbelievable size. It was extremely painful and incredibly ugly. My nose looked twice its size. I was thirteen years old.

Over the years, the cold sores became more and more prevalent. They spread down my nose, onto my upper lip, into my nose, and all over my lips. Still, today, I fight them, and it is rare that I do not have at least one at all times.

My period started when I was ten or eleven and they were incredibly heavy. I would wear the most absorbent tampon with the thickest pad. My classes were forty-five minutes long, and I found myself running to the bathroom after each class to change both the tampon and the pad. Many times, I would have blood running down my legs. This would go on for seven to ten days every month.

By fourteen or fifteen, I was struggling with the normal things a girl that age struggles with; boys, friends, clothes, make-up. But I had a few extra concerns. I found I had severe mood swings.

My relationships with friends were always very volatile. I would come home crying to my mom every day. She would sit for hours and try to calm me. I remember her taking me to the mall, and we would walk through the stores and talk. She had such a soothing way of handling my fifteen-year-old problems. I always felt so safe and secure with her.

I would explain to my mom that I would be talking to someone at school and having a very normal conversation when suddenly, without warning, a severe mood change would hit me and I would start screaming. I would hover above myself and watch as I lost complete control over my behavior, and as I hovered, I would be thinking, *Stop, stop-why won't you stop?*

But my emotions were completely out of control and I could not stop.

Soon, it became apparent these mood swings were far worse that just an emotional teen acting out. It was clear I needed help. My mom took me to the gynecologist for my first Pap smear. During the office visit, she explained to the doctor that if something were not done soon, I would be homicidal. The doctor laughed and corrected her by saying,

"You mean suicidal?"

She said, "No, homicidal. She'll kill someone one day."

The doctor explained the benefits of putting me on the birth control pill. He felt this might not only slow down my periods, and cause me to bleed less, but it should stabilize my moods. I was fifteen years old.

Very shortly after starting the pill, I found I was much calmer. Not only were my moods less erratic, but my periods were much easier. I did not bleed as much, I was not scream-ing at everyone I saw, I did not cry as often, and I did not have to find new friends every month. Life was becoming easier.

Things that would set me off before did not bother me any more.

In high school, shortly after starting the pill, I was assigned an essay entitled "Who are you?" I wrote the best essay I could — considering all of the amazing changes taking place. My teacher called me up after class, and said this essay was not of the quality I had turned in before. I remember breaking down, crying and saying "But I don't know who I am."

Even though these changes were wonderful and freeing, I still found it difficult to relate to myself. At fifteen years old, I was starting over. Like teen-dom was not hard enough. My teacher, sensing the extreme stress this was causing, inquired, "Why don't you write about that?"

I think it was one of the best essays I have written, and from then on, I found myself a little more bearable. I started to understand who I was. In fact, I started to actually like who I was becoming.

At seventeen I was in a severe car accident. The witnesses swore the driver — me — had been killed. Surprisingly, I walked away. My mom took me to a doctor that afternoon to be checked, and he found I was all right.

Within a matter of days, I was having severe back pain, dizziness, and was starting to miss classes. My mom's co-worker's son was a chiropractor, and recommended I make an appointment. I saw him for some time, and slowly, my back improved.

While in treatment, I started to notice a lump on the right side of my neck. It was up under my jaw, so I am sure my parents thought it was a lymph node. It grew quickly, and became about the size of a golf ball.

I went to a doctor, and he decided to do a test on the salivary gland. He believed it might be blocked or infected. I was told the test was no big deal; all they would do is inject dye into the gland and then take x-rays. I remember being petrified because they were going to stick a needle through my neck.

My dad took me to the hospital, and I was so scared. I went into this sterile room, and sat on a huge x-ray table. The doctor came in and put on a headlamp. He seemed to have some trouble and played around with it for a few moments. An assistant finally came over, took it off of his head, turned it over, and put it back on with a perfect fit.

"Doctor, you had it on upside down," he said. The fear I already felt became terror.

The procedure involved injecting dye with a cannula inserted into the salivary gland opening in my mouth and a few x-rays. There was, fortunately, no pain, but there would also be no resolution to my problem. The salivary gland was normal. Within a few months, the swelling had reduced, and the situation was forgotten.

Not too long after the swollen gland, I developed a severe sinus infection. I was given a shot of Demerol for pain. I remember as I was telling my mom the shot would not affect me, my body went quite limp and my speech slurred. I kind of remember my parent's carrying me to bed. After that, I remember waking up to go to the bathroom in the middle of the night and when I went back to bed, I was so weak, I fell to my knees and started crawling back to room. My mom heard me, and I remember her helping me.

During my senior year of high school, my family took a trip to England. A few days after returning home, I broke out with what was believed to be the chicken pox. I had small red blisters all over my body, and because I never had them, a doctor assumed the diagnosis.

I found that all through high school, I slept. I would come home from school, and sleep for about three hours. I'd wake up and eat, and then go to bed that night for twelve hours. The doctors said I would grow out of it. After all, I was a teenager and needed extra sleep because I was growing. But they were wrong; I never grew out of it. And I never stopped sleeping.

I continued to experience small ups and downs throughout my teens and early twenties. Most illnesses would be considered normal in and of themselves, but as I look back and reflect on the whole picture, I can't help but wonder how all of the small problems have contributed to the big issue I face now as an adult.

Did a doctor miss something?

Should I have done something different?

So many questions have raced through my head over the years. Unfortunately, I have realized I will never know the answers.

Diagnosis

*M*y search for a diagnosis was long and exhausting. I struggled with my health for a dozen years before a doctor not only believed me, but also acknowledged my symptoms.

Over the years, people have questioned my need for a diagnosis, and cannot understand why I have gone from doctor to doctor to find answers. They are unable to understand why I do not just accept that no one knows what is wrong with me.

Diagnosing people with CFIDS can be highly beneficial but tremendously destructive. On one hand, I could finally give my suffering a name, but on the other hand, it is a "catch-all" diagnosis. The doctors did not know how else to explain my myriad of symptoms.

By giving the disease and the problem a name, I felt as if I was being validated. I felt like the medical community was accepting me. By giving my disease a name, it gave me something to fight. I could define my enemy. I now had my own personal crusade. I thought it would allow me to form a plan of attack. Until now, I was shooting in the dark. I had no direction. How do you fight something you cannot identify? How do you fight when nobody believes you?

Unfortunately, those initial hopeful feelings were soon shattered. The more I learned, the more scared I became. I had a diagnosis, but what did that accomplish? I was still sick. I still had no cure. I still did not know what it meant to have CFIDS. Unfortunately, my future was looking just as bleak as before I had a name for my disease.

The first hurdle had been overcome, but the hurdles ahead were looking taller, and more foreboding than ever.

At the time of my diagnosis, I was twenty-four years old and living at home. I was in school, and working at an emergency animal hospital when I started to have very severe fatigue problems. I was sleeping most of the time and finding I was having trouble getting through the day without feeling like I was going to collapse. My work started to suffer, and I found that my concentration skills were fading.

My mom knew a woman whose husband was a doctor. He found CFIDS challenging, and was showing an interest in working with those who were afflicted with the devastating disease. With very little hope, I made an appointment. If anything, I figured I might find a sympathetic ear.

I arrived at my first appointment thinking, *Here we go, I'll have to explain the whole thing — AGAIN!* But this doctor was different. When he came into the room, I did not feel like I had to justify myself. He put me at ease immediately. He had a sort of mad scientist/Patch Adams quality. I was able to explain what I was going through without feeling embarrassed. He showed me, for the first time, some compassion and he listened without judging. Whether he believed me or not, he treated me with respect and took my complaints seriously.

He talked to me about a disease called Chronic Fatigue Syndrome and the relationship it bears to the Epstein-Barr virus — the belief at the time. He wanted to run the EBV panel and do full blood work.

He also talked to me about depression. He was not worried

about clinical depression, or depression causing my symptoms, but felt I might become depressed because I could not muster enough energy to get out of bed every day. He asked me to consider starting the anti-depressant drug Prozac so we could ward off any depression that might contribute to the fatigue.

He felt keeping my spirits up would keep the disease from becoming worse. I decided to think about starting the medication. After I had the blood results, I could make a more informed decision. I had my blood drawn and went home to anxiously await the findings.

My recheck was a week later. During that time, I fought the idea of going on an anti-depressant, especially Prozac. I was familiar with all the horror stories involving the drug, and I was afraid. My parents were not keen on the idea, but the more we talked about it, the fear of getting worse convinced me to try it.

I went back to the doctor and he told me my EBV test showed not only exposure, which most of the population will show — but also activity. This was quite rare, and he considered sending me to an infectious disease specialist.

He explained that the EBV is responsible for mononucleosis in teenagers, but was concerned because I was in my mid-twenties. He felt the most appropriate diagnosis was CFIDS. He wanted to try an extremely strong dose of anti-virals and see if it would make any difference in my lab values. I told him I had decided to start on Prozac and I left the office with the two prescriptions.

As I walked out of the building, I began to cry. I sat in my car for about ten minutes and sobbed. I felt an uncontrollable wave of despair and fear. I finally let out twelve years of frustration and anger. I was devastated, how could this happen to me? What had I done to deserve this? And why had it taken SO long to get to this point?

When I arrived home, my parents were anxiously waiting. The look on my face and my red swollen eyes told them it was not good news. I told them I have the Epstein-Barr Virus, and the assumption was that I have CFIDS. Through tears, I explained the anti-viral trial and the Prozac.

My mom cried and my dad was at a loss for words. They were flabbergasted and devastated. After what seemed like an hour of silence from both my parents, and endless stifled sobs from me, my mom wiped her eyes, smiled, put her arms around me, and said, "Well, we finally know what it is, now it's time to fight!"

In a whisper I cried, "But I'm so tired, Mom, I don't think I can." My voice quivered and my words were almost inaudible.

"Then we'll just have to do it for you," she proclaimed with all the confidence of a mother bear protecting one of her beloved cubs. At that moment, she had nothing but courage.

I had some difficulty adjusting to the Prozac. My dosing was small in the beginning and then slowly increased over the next month. I had some dizzy spells and slight nausea at first, but I felt a lessening of my symptoms eventually.

I took the anti-virals as directed, and returned to have the EBV test re-run. This time, it showed past activity, but no current infection. The doctor felt as though the problem was basically solved, and sent me home with instructions to re-check if I was not feeling well. Unfortunately, CFIDS does not just "go away" — and the problem would not be that simple to solve.

My mom had her new mission; she was fighting for her daughter's life. She was done sitting idly by while my strength and spirit were being sucked from my body. However, her fight quickly became discouraging. The little bit of information she found was disheartening. The help out there was scarce and bleak. She scoured newspapers and magazines for anything helping fatigue, and we tried everything we saw.

Mineral supplements and herbal concoctions were the most popular. CFIDS was starting to be recognized and the supplement companies were jumping on the bandwagon. Unfortunately, none of these remedies helped my case. The Prozac was in full effect within a couple of months. I started to feel less fatigued, but underlying exhaustion was always present. My mental outlook became brighter, but I was still plagued with tremendous fear. My diagnosis became a little easier to handle. I continued to work and live my life despite the fatigue I felt every day. We believed it was under control. And it was — for the moment.

My Career Path

$\mathcal{I}$ wanted to be a veterinarian from the time I could speak. Working with animals was the only thing I could imagine myself doing. In grade school, we would list our top three choices for careers when we grew up. The teachers would get so frustrated with me because I would put veterinarian on all three lines.

There was no other option for me. I would not even entertain the thought of doing something else. With that assumption in mind, my mom asked the veterinarian down the street if I would be able to clean cages for him or do various odd jobs around the hospital.

I was only fourteen at the time, and he said I would have to be at least sixteen to work. He invited me to come by sometime and watch a surgery, or spend some time in the clinic to see if I was truly interested in veterinary medicine.

I decided to go in one afternoon and watch a dog neuter. My friend went with me. We walked into the surgical suite, and stood next to the door. The room was very sterile, and the dog lay on his back, spread eagle, with his legs tied down on all four sides of the stainless steel table. There was a tube sticking out of the dog's mouth, and the groin area had been shaved.

The doctor entered the room and put on gloves, a gown, and a mask. He picked up his scalpel, and made a small incision along the scrotum. He squeezed beneath the testicle, and it popped out of the opening.

He grabbed the pink, round ball of flesh, pulled it straight up and tore the ligaments that held it close to the body. By releasing the ligaments, he was able to pull the testicle about two to three inches from the body. From there he was able to use the scalpel to cut the final vessels holding the testicle in place.

I had never been faint or passed out in my life, but I felt this strange sense of heat and nausea come over me. I walked out of the room and down the hallway, back into the waiting area. I sat down, put my head down to my knees, and tried to take some deep breaths. Surprisingly enough, my friend, who was known for her weak stomach, stayed and watched the whole procedure.

I went home and decided this veterinarian thing was not so appealing after all. Who would of thought such things were done? I had no idea. I thought that I would be giving animals love and affection. Instead, I was going to be torturing them! I tucked the experience away and continued living my life, all along realizing veterinary medicine was probably not for me.

I soon found that make-up, clothes and boys were more interesting than worrying about what terrible things I might have to do to animals.

My oldest brother worked at Nordstrom as the stock boy in the cosmetic department. He was able to get me a job during the Christmas of my fifteenth year as the cosmetic gift wrapper. I was at a table in the middle of the department, and I would wrap the perfume that men bought for their wives and girlfriends.

It was so glamorous and I loved every minute of it. The women that worked there were all so pretty and graceful. I decided then and there that I wanted to be a cosmetics sales-girl. I started to practice applying make-up and experiment-ed with different products and potions.

Nordstrom had started it's own teen line of cosmetics called Colour Etc., and I was one of the first girls on the list to represent it. I was sixteen and selling cosmetics at one of the top department stores on the West Coast. I soon found, though, I was not a very good saleswoman. I found myself trying so hard to educate people I would forget to close the sale. But it was a great experience, and I really liked the industry.

In the car one day, my mom and I were talking about my grades, and she said if I wanted to get into UC Davis for veterinary school, I had better get my grades up. Otherwise, I should start considering a new career path.

Without any hesitation and no argument I said, "Okay, I want to go into the cosmetic industry."

My mom and dad always supported my every whim — and with this new career goal in mind, they had me find out what I needed to do to make it happen.

I decided I wanted to do make-up for magazine covers. I thought it would be exciting. After some thought, I realized the cosmetic and fashion industry seemed to be based in Europe. So the summer of my junior year in high school, my family took a vacation to England. While there, I interviewed at two of the top cosmetology schools. The head mistress said they would prefer not to have me come when I was so young, but they would not completely rule out an application based on age.

We finished our trip and on the way home, I realized there had to be schools like this in California. After all, Los Angeles was a top fashion center as well.

I started to do some research, and found the Fashion Institute of Design and Merchandising (FIDM). Better yet, my first year would be in Orange County, and the second year in Los Angeles. I went to an interview and found that most of the courses were fashion-related.

I quickly became discouraged because my focus was cosmetics, but the counselor explained they might have something of interest and I should call back in one week.

A week later, I called and learned they had started a major called Cosmetic and Fragrance Merchandise Marketing. They had the final meeting to approve it on the day I came in to interview. I was the first student accepted into the program. I could not believe what a perfect opportunity. I attended every class and couldn't wait to get up in the morning to go to school.

I obtained a prized job as an Estee Lauder cosmetic salesgirl at The Broadway department store at eighteen years old, and was one of their youngest salesgirls. Unfortunately, my sales skills were, at best, marginal and I struggled with quotas and goals.

From there, I went back to Nordstrom and worked for Erno Laszlo skincare. I deeply believed in the product, but I could not relate to the older clientele. I heard women say repeatedly that I could not understand aging because I was so young.

In many ways they were right. My sales were poor and the buyers and account managers were not pleased with my performance. For the first time in my life, I was not the best.

I graduated from FIDM at twenty years old and decided to try a different road. I found a job with a company called Draper's & Damon's. They had multiple stores on the West Coast and a catalog that carried clothing for the mature women. I became the assistant buyer of women's sportswear and had a tough-as-nails boss. I not only admired her deeply, but I worked very hard to make her proud of me.

I soon proved I was an exceptional employee and was placed in charge of the catalog sportswear division. It was my responsibility to monitor and analyze sales of specific catalog items and re-order the merchandise so we did not run out of stock. I did this for more than two years and then found I was growing bored. I had mastered the job, and the challenge was gone. People started commenting that I should try to model, and I decided to try my hand at it.

At twenty-one years old I was hired as a Budweiser girl and a Jagermeister girl. I would go to bars in very little clothing and promote the liquor. I did various appearances and poster signings. I worked at golf tournaments and special events. I was one of the lucky ones who appeared on the poster.

It was the first time I felt really popular. I would walk into a bar, and every man there wanted to talk to me. At the time, I did not care that the attention was negative; I learned to keep my focus on what it really was. I never dated anyone I met at the bars and I knew that the only reason I was getting all of that attention was because I was not wearing very much clothing. But, never the less, it still made me feel good.

I started to be recognized outside of the uniform. I would go to a bar on my off time, and people would say, "That's the Bud girl!"

It was so exciting, I was a mini celebrity — I loved it.

The amazing part of the whole thing is that I didn't drink. Not a drop! I would get such bad headaches; it was not worth it. I was also very shy, but when I put on that uniform, I became someone else. I could be whomever I wanted. I could hide behind my body. I had all the self-confidence in the world, but the minute that uniform came off, I found myself to be shy and self-conscience.

I quit my job at Draper's & Damon's and started to put my modeling portfolio together. I blossomed in front of the camera. I took acting lessons and was a natural. I loved being in front of the camera, and I loved the attention.

Unfortunately, my health was starting to slowly deteriorate. I took my portfolio to a few agents, and was almost laughed out of their offices. They always said I was not what they were looking for. One said my lips were too big, another said they were too thin. My chest was too big for one, and too small for the other.

I did some extra work for the movies, but I couldn't maintain the long hours. I tried an infomercial, but have never seen it. I hated the rejection, and resented the way it made me feel.

I could not take it with a grain of salt and move on. The constant criticism did not just roll off my back. It quickly became clear I was too sensitive to be in show business.

To make ends meet, I started waiting tables at a pool hall.

My mom and I went to lunch one day, and as we were sitting in the restaurant eating lunch, I started to cry. I told her I was sick of being judged on my looks — to have someone decide my value based on my body. I knew there was more to life.

I decided I needed to get back to basics — to find what truly made me happy. I loved animals and there had to be something I could do in this field. We had just recently had my childhood dog euthanized and the hospital we went to was amazing. It was almost better than any human facility I had ever been to. I applied for a job and was hired on the spot.

I found out that there was a nursing school for animals, and I enrolled immediately. Once again, I was a top student — and I could not learn fast enough.

I was quickly put into the Critical Care Unit at the hospital, and worked with the most critically ill patients. My supervisor took me under her wing and acted as my mentor. I learned so much from her. I continued to work for the alcohol companies while in school. It was easy money, and I could choose my hours.

But while in school, I started having severe problems with my health. I began taking Prozac and gradually gained a tremendous amount of weight.

Because of my increasing size, my job with the alcohol companies came to an end. It was a sign letting me know they judged me strictly on my appearance and not my sales performance.

I finished school, and sat for my state boards. I passed and became Stephanie Kelley, R.V.T. (Registered Veterinary Technician). I was a great nurse, with exceptional skills, and unending compassion. Quitting my job with the alcohol companies was no longer considered a loss. I finally found something that really made me feel good about myself.

After I finished school, I decided to move to San Diego. My best friend and her family were there, and their next-door neighbor rented me a room. I got a job at an emergency hospital close by and enjoyed my time there. My health caused me to move home after only three months — and I was unable to work for some time.

When I was well enough to go back to work, I was hired at a new specialty animal hospital that had recently been opened. I had worked for the owner at an emergency hospital before I moved to San Diego and really respected him as a veterinarian.

He had seen how CFIDS had affected my life and always found the ability to show me compassion and concern. The head technician also knew my history, but respected how hard I worked and knew I was a skilled nurse. I was fortunate enough to be hired within the first few months of opening the business. I enjoyed the new challenge of helping to build this blossoming practice, and I worked extremely hard.

The veterinarian who owned the practice had a tremendous reputation throughout the community, and our cages were always full with exciting and interesting cases. I quickly became the supervisor, and oversaw a shift of five to six technicians. I had also taken over the monthly billing, and handled all of the client inquiries, and complaints relating to their invoices.

The owner worked hard to show his staff as much appreciation as possible, and the staff turnover was minimal. As far as veterinary hospitals go, he was a superior employer.

Once again, life was moving along beautifully. But one morning, I woke up and something was different.

That familiar feeling of exhaustion overcame me. I went to work that afternoon, and felt progressively worse. I pushed to finish my shift, and made it through the evening. The next day, I again got up and went to work. This time, though, I commented to my friend that I wasn't sure if I would be able to finish my shift.

I continued to work for another hour or so, and my friend approached me to find out how I was doing. I was holding undeveloped x-rays in my arms, and explaining how sick I was feeling when the owner of the practice walked up and started to ask my friend for some assistance with a patient. He looked at me, and immediately recognized something was wrong.

"Are you okay?" he asked.

I started to cry and my friend told him I was sick.

He nonchalantly looked at me and said, "Well then, go home. We're all right."

"No, you don't understand," I could barely say the next few words, "I'm getting sick again." Tears flowed slowly down my face, and I looked at the ground — I could not look him in the eye. Once again I was embarrassed and scared.

It took a split second for him to comprehend the implications of our brief interaction that afternoon, and obvious concern and sadness washed over his face. I quickly walked away from them and went into the darkroom to develop the x-rays. As I opened the door, the owner was standing outside.

He put his arm around me, and said, "You do what you need to do, your health is the most important thing right now."

"But I'll be letting everyone down," I said, wiping the tears from my eyes and making a weak attempt to stand tall, causing him to remove his arm from my shoulder. It was a pathetic effort to show a courageous front. I wanted him to believe I was over my moment of weakness, and I was fine now. I needed to get back to work, and I made a slight movement forward in an effort to walk past him.

Quickly, he maneuvered himself in front of me, put both hands on my shoulders, looked me square in the eye, and said firmly, "So what? GO HOME!"

He did not fall for my lousy show of bravado.

I immediately started to cry, thanked him in barely a whisper, and told him I would be in touch with the office manager to find out what to do from here.

The next day I called the hospital administrator, and found that the owner had already been to see her. He had told her that no matter what happens to Stephanie, she would always have a job at his hospital.

I felt an immediate and tremendous sense of relief. We worked out a schedule where I came in three days a week for three hours at a time and worked on billing issues. I could increase my hours at any time and the manager explained she had a number of projects she could give me. This way, I would never be without work.

It was perfect. I kept my job, but was able to work around my illness.

Everyone was shocked I was sick. I had not told anyone I suffered from CFIDS. When I saw the head technician, I apologized for the quick departure from the hospital floor.

His comment to me was simply, "Hey, we knew this could happen when we hired you. It's no problem."

I would drag myself to work three times a week, and never complained. In fact, the year I worked this way, I never called out sick. I left early a handful of times, but I was so grateful for the ability to keep my job I never "played on" my struggle.

I worked hard while I was there, and always tried to be helpful and cheerful. Occasionally, I would explain to a co-worker, who showed interest, how hard life was when I was sick. The universal response was, "I had no idea you were going through that."

Through it all, the owner of the practice continued to work with me so I did not have to leave. Finally, as I wrote this book, I put in my final notice. My husband and I were ready to pursue other interests. On my last day, it took forty-five minutes to say good-bye to the all the people I had been with for two and a half years.

By far, the hardest good-bye was the owner. I cried the minute I walked over to him. He had always been modest, and I obviously made him uncomfortable, but I had to thank him for all the support and love he had shown me over the last few years. He never looked me in the eye as I spoke, but the last thing he said to me was, "Thank you for all you've done for me."

I'll never forget his compassion. It would have been easy to fire me or never hire me to begin with, but he is one of the few genuinely good people in this world. And for that, he will always hold a special place in my heart, and I am honored to consider him a friend.

With that, my career with animals ended. I have wondered, recently, if my exposure to chemicals and animals has contributed to my poor health. I had never been completely bedridden until I started working in hospitals. Could that be the link?

I do miss working with animals, though. My passion was emergency and critical care. It was incredibly rewarding and I felt as though I made a difference. In a strange way, I have had to mourn the loss of a true love.

At this point, I am afraid to become involved in any aspect of the animal field again. I truly believe there is some sort of connection with my declining health.

The anesthesia I would breathe everyday, radiation I was constantly being exposed to, chemicals, urine, and dander I was always in contact with... the possibilities are limitless. Could one — or a combination of all of those things — be the reason I have suffered so much grief over the years?

For now, away from animals, I take one day at a time. Some are good; some not so good. But, to date, I have not been nearly as sick as before. I also pace myself better now. I do not work ten to twelve hour days. I do not force myself to push harder. And, I guess only time will tell if I found what exacerbates my CFIDS.

You Weigh What?!

*A*fter starting Prozac, I found myself facing a real dilemma. I was feeling more energized, but my weight was becoming a real problem. I was a slim and trim 110 pounds when I started the medication, but during the first year, I packed on sixty pounds.

Like many people on anti-depressants, I became lost in the medical system and, for four years, I took Prozac every morning. Eventually my weight was pushing 200 pounds. As scary as the weight gain was, I was more terrified to stop the medication. I was emotionally satisfied, and my health was reasonably stable, so I overlooked the weight. After all, being overweight was a small price to pay for not being in bed every day.

My job with Jagermeister began to suffer. I bought and wore snug pants instead of the cute short skirts I was wearing before. My sales were high, but I knew my physical appearance was still of top priority. It did not matter whether I was good at selling the product, I did not look the part anymore, and the security of my job was jeopardized. For the first time in my life, I was insecure about my body.

My final promotion was at a bar in Long Beach, California. It started like any other. We usually worked in pairs, but the bar was so small they could not justify sending two girls. When I arrived, I parked on the side street and entered the building from the front.

The room the bar was in did not look much bigger than a small storefront in a strip mall. The walls were covered with beer posters displaying half-naked women playfully holding bottles. Neon signs screamed at customers to try this beer or that. People were crammed into every corner and lined the counter of the horseshoe shaped bar in the middle of the room. The lights were dim, the air was dingy, and the jukebox screamed some old rock and roll tune.

I walked through the entrance of the bar and all heads turned and looked at me. I could feel the eyes of men, and women, following me as I made my way through the tight-knit crowd. It was as if all of these local people were questioning whom this stranger was invading their private space. Local bars were always the same. Initially, patrons were on guard, but they quickly warmed up and welcomed us with open arms.

The open end of the horseshoe bar led into a back storeroom. After talking with the manager, I went to the storeroom, and took a few moments to get ready. Finally, I walked out into the bar and quickly assessed the crowd.

Each bar had its own personality, and it was important to plan your strategy around it. I did not think I could occupy two hours by just socializing with the small number of clientele so I thought it would be fun to get behind the bar and ask trivia questions for Jagermeister prizes. I decided to walk around the room and interact directly with the patrons for an hour and a half, then during the last half-hour or so, I would do the contest.

I walked around for a little while and enjoyed chatting with the customers. Then, as planned, I went behind the bar. The manager got everyone's attention and the customers all huddled around the counter so they could hear me and vie for their shot at a Jagermeister shirt. I started asking various trivia type questions.

"What does Jagermeister mean?"

"How many herbs and spices are in Jagermeister?"

"Who sings the song playing on the jukebox right now?"

This continued for approximately fifteen minutes and people seemed to really enjoy playing for Jagermeister merchandise.

However, one guy decided he had had enough.

"Aren't you too fat to be a Jagermeister girl?" wafted through the air and endlessly echoed in my ears.

The crowd fell silent. I was horrified, hurt, mad, and humiliated — all at the same time. After what seemed like an hour, a low buzz crept through the bar and my mind assumed that everyone agreed with this drunk. All these people who were having so much fun seconds before, now agreed that I was too fat for this job.

I summoned every ounce of inner strength I could find; asked one more question, thanked the manager and immediately left.

As I practically ran out of the bar, I swore I heard, "Wow! She really is fat!" from the people I passed.

The second I hit the fresh air, the tears began to well up in my eyes. I sat in my car and sobbed.

I cried all the way home. Fortunately I arrived home late, and my parents were already asleep. There was no one to question my swollen eyes. I called my boss the next day. I explained that with my regular job and school, I was far too busy to continue doing promotions. She said she was sorry to hear I was quitting, but I should call when I was ready to pick-up more shifts.

She obviously had not seen me recently, or the offer would not have been made. I never spoke of that night in the bar. I was too humiliated.

Occasionally, I would look at my modeling portfolio, and see this small firm body. A sense of despair would wash over me, but my trusted friend Prozac kept me from dwelling on what I had become. Every time I looked at those pictures, I would vow to start dieting and working out the next morning. But the next morning would come and go — and I still found myself too tired to care.

The hardest part was fighting with my cravings. I had never had food issues, and have not since I have been off Prozac, but the drug altered the chemistry in my brain. I had to have certain foods.

I worked the swing shift and would, at times, get off work at three or four o'clock in the morning. I would find myself at the grocery store buying chocolate chip cookies. I had no control. It was as if my car would drive itself to the store. I had no recollection of the drive, and would suddenly become aware while I was paying at the register. By then, though, it was too late. My course, that night, was set. I needed to binge.

I would fill an extra large coffee mug to the rim with cookies and saturate it with milk. Within twenty minutes, the bag was gone and I was feeling more disgusted with myself than ever. I loved canned frosting and again, I would sit in front of the TV, and eat the whole can. My meals consisted of canned spaghetti and chips.

I found myself bingeing when I was alone. I was too scared to do it in front of people. They might confront me, and I would lose the one thing I thought I had control of. I was always so disgusted with myself, but I could not stop. In my desperate attempt to control something in my life, I actually lost my self-respect and dignity.

Many evenings I would decide to start dieting and exercising the next morning. But, by ten the next morning, I was bingeing again.

I was never able to purge. I could not allow myself to cross that line. Besides, I hate throwing up when I am sick, so the idea of doing it on purpose horrifies me.

I could never discount the complete escape food offered me. It never doubted my illness; never questioned the validity of my symptoms, and it gave me the comfort I needed.

I had no control over my health at this point, and there were no treatments on the horizon. Food was my treatment, and for that brief instant while I was eating, it worked.

My family noticed this physical change, but focusing on weight was never popular in their house. They loved me, and my weight did not matter. But I am sure they would have thought differently had they known what I was doing to myself.

It quickly became clear that I would need new clothes and this ritual repeated itself every six months. I hated shopping because the mirrors in the dressing room laughed at me, and I knew the sales girls were mocking me when they said how great I looked. I bought anything that covered my increasing size.

My days of crop tops and short skirts were over. I avoided anything form fitting; the baggier the better. It was easy to hide behind cargo pants and sweatshirts. This way, no one could see how big I really was.

Within a few years, I was busting out of size eighteen, and getting ready to buy size twenty. I had trouble walking up stairs and accomplishing daily tasks. Not only was my fatigue severe enough to cause me to stop and catch my breath at the slightest exertion, but carrying almost a hundred pounds of extra weight was exhausting me too.

I would sit in a chair, and I could not cross my legs. It was difficult, if not impossible to wear shorts or a dress, because my upper thighs would rub together and cause terrible blistering, and severe chaffing. My hips had become so wide it was hard to wear jeans, they just did not fit right. Through it all, I still maintained a relatively small waist and in order to find pants that fit my hips, the waistband would be huge.

My hipbones ached and my knees screamed. I experienced heart palpitations and would almost pass out when I stood up. My heart was working overtime trying to pump blood through my enormous body. I gained the weight so fast my body did not have time to accommodate the ever-increasing stress I was inflicting on it.

During one of my healthier times, my friend thought it would be fun to walk a marathon for a charitable organization. She asked if I was interested and I agreed to go to the orientation meeting. I was not ready to commit, but throughout the meeting I remember thinking not only was this a wonderful cause, but what an amazing personal triumph. I would prove to CFIDS, once and for all, that I was in control. I decided to join the team that night.

Shortly after the orientation, we went to a pep rally where we were introduced to people who suffered from the disease the charity helped. I was inspired to see how all of these victims were not really victims at all. They were happy and spirited — and tried to live life to the fullest. Even in the face of tragedy they seemed to be happy to be alive.

After the meeting, my friend and I went out into the hallway for our weigh-in and body fat check. The organization wanted us to succeed, and they were prepared to help us along the way. I stepped on the scale, and felt a sense of horror. The weight read 192, and the body fat started blinking thirty-eight per cent.

The muscular hunk in charge of the weigh-in looked at me very callously and said, "Wow, thirty-eight percent body fat, you're clinically obese!"

Once again, I was mortified. Yet sadly, I was totally powerless against my ever-increasing size. The training began and consisted of long walks. Over many months, distance was added and endurance was increased. From the beginning, I found excuses to avoid the training sessions and within two months, I dropped out due to my declining health. My personal triumph became a huge defeat. CFIDS won again, and I never did complete a marathon.

About two years ago, a doctor observed that I was not showing signs of depression. He advised me it was time to go off Prozac. I was both terrified and excited at the same time. I knew, in the back of my mind, I would lose weight. But my emotional stability was at stake. I decided the benefits were worth the risk and after four years, I took my final pill.

Shortly after stopping the medication, I remember thinking, *Where'd my appetite go?* I suddenly did not feel this obsessive need to eat. I was not feeling the uncontrollable cravings. I could eat one or two cookies — and not an entire package. I felt sane again and my emotions were remaining stable.

Within the first three months of stopping the drug, I dropped twenty-five pounds without effort. My boyfriend and I decided to do an intense weight loss and exercise program. I committed completely. During the four months of the program I lost an additional forty pounds. When all was said and done, I had lost seventy pounds in less than a year.

I felt healthier and happier and was looking forward to my "new" life. But sadly, CFIDS did not care about my incredible weight loss story. It did not care if I was 200 or 135 pounds. It could still lash out at any time. It could still make its presence known. And just when I thought it had left for good it would attack again with all its might.

A Change of Pace

*T*had been having problems with my health for many years, but had always been able to live a reasonably full life. I was working a full time job in an emergency animal hospital. I also had a second part time job with Jagermeister and Budweiser, and attended school full time to become a registered veterinary nurse.

I was burning the candle at both ends, and in the process becoming burned out. Toward the end of my schooling I was itching for a change of pace. I had recently quit Jagermeister due to my weight gain, and I did not have anything keeping me in Orange County.

My friend, Ann, and her family lived in San Diego, and I always loved being there. San Diego's atmosphere was always so laid back and the people were always so nice. It was the epitome of a beach town.

I called Ann and told her I was moving to her hometown. She was not only thrilled, but also explained how her next-door neighbor, who was a young schoolteacher, was looking for another roommate.

The house was brand new, and the neighbor had already rented one of the rooms in her three-bedroom place.

I called the neighbor later that day and we hit it off immediately. We made plans to meet that weekend. To make the most of the trip to San Diego, I also set up an interview with a hospital in the area. A friend at my current job referred me to the hospital he used to work for while he lived in San Diego. In fact, he called the hospital and gave me a glowing recommendation. The interview itself was mostly a formality, because I was pretty much offered the job over the phone.

My parents and I drove down to San Diego that weekend and saw both the house and the hospital. Both situations were perfect for me, and I put a security deposit down for the house, and accepted the job. On Wednesday of the next week, I took my last final exam at school, and by Friday I was moving to San Diego.

My parents and brother helped me and we were able to complete the move in one trip.

The house was great. I had my own room, and shared the bathroom with the other tenant. Outside of our rooms was a small sitting area where I put my entertainment center with a TV and stereo. The owner of the house had an extra couch we put in the room as well. Downstairs was a nice living room, big kitchen, and small dining room. It was a great house!

Within a day or two I started my new job, and loved it. Everyone was kind, and I hit it off with my now-best-friend, Jennifer. We became instant companions because we had a common ground. We both suffered from chronic illness and found peace when we were with each other.

We were able to talk, for the first time, about the feelings and internal pain associated with our respective diseases. Jennifer suffered from bulimia and anorexia, and had struggled since she was twelve years old. Even though she still fought, and at times failed, with the urge to binge and purge, I was impressed with her inner strength. She still had a sense of peace about her.

Jennifer had survived a suicide attempt, had been hospitalized for the damage she had caused, and needed her gums repaired because of the stomach acids destroying her mouth. This was a constant and ongoing battle she fought, but I always felt a sense of calm around her.

Jennifer was very thin; although I know in her mind she believed she was overweight. Her hair was incredibly long, down to her waist, and amazingly thick. She was absolutely beautiful, both inside and out. Her kindness was apparent to everyone in her presence — and it was hard not to fall in love with her. She was mild-mannered, gentle, and very soft-spoken.

I started to learn all of the internal battles Jennifer fought every day, and she learned mine. She never judged me; only treated me with a compassion I have never felt before. I realized for the first time how a friend could understand what my life was like.

I worked the swing shift while in San Diego, and would not get home until after two in the morning most nights. I regret that I was not able to spend more time with my friend, Ann, and her family. After all, she was right next door. But she was busy with her two children, her husband, and her brand new house. I was also sleeping most of the mornings and afternoons, so I would be fresh for the night shifts. We really lived our lives at different times of the day.

I will always remember, though, Ann's husband building a new patio in their backyard. I would work a twelve-hour shift and not get to bed until four a.m. By ten that morning, I would jump out of bed — scared to death by an automatic paint sprayer. The noise was deafening and so annoying. There was no possible way to sleep through it.

Her husband would be pounding and painting away, and my window was about twenty feet from his workspace. To this day, I still tease them about it.

The times I did spend with Ann and her family were wonderful. Since they had lived so far away for so long, it was nice to be able to just walk out the front door and have them so close.

For about three months, I continued to work and try to start my life in San Diego. The house I lived in was empty most of the time. The two girls were always gone and would stay with friends many nights. When they were at home, our schedules conflicted, so I was not able to develop a friendship with either of them. This made for a very easy living situation, but now I kind of regret not making more of an effort to get to know them.

I was developing some friendships at work, but I rarely went out, and found I was very shy in such a foreign situation. It was very difficult, and still is difficult, for me to make friends. I never felt well enough to cultivate and work at a relationship.

Realizing I had to get out of the house to meet people, I started to do things on my own. I bought a pass to Sea World, and would go on my days off. I would spend a couple of hours there, and would usually spend most of my time with the manatees. Occasionally I would see a show, but the manatee exhibit was my favorite.

I would sit for an hour or more, and just watch them. They were so sad, they moved so slow, and I remember hearing people say how ugly they were as they stood and watched them. I guess I felt a feeling of oneness with them. I could sympathize with their plight. I knew the sadness I saw in their eyes.

I always found manatees beautiful and graceful — and my heart always broke when I would hear the stories about the boats hitting them. This ritual created a peace for me. I really enjoyed the time I spent at Sea World, and it kept me busy.

I had been in San Diego for about three months when I woke up one morning and felt different. For the first time, I was not sure if I could continue to work.

I called my parents, and told them that I thought I was getting really sick. Granted, I had been sick in the past, but this was different. It was all consuming. My entire body felt like it was shutting down.

My mom told me to wait until the weekend, and do not do anything until they came. They both worked and could not just run down on a whim.

The more we talked, the more they realized how sick I was. They both got the next day off and planned to come down to see me so we could figure out what to do next. My mom encouraged me to pull myself together and get through work that night. Through tears, I told her I would and I would see them tomorrow.

I dragged myself into work, and while assisting in surgery with one of the veterinarians, I explained my situation and told him I may not be able to work any longer. He understood, and told me to do whatever I needed to do.

That night, I tried to focus on work, but I would look at a treatment chart and have no idea what it was. It was as if I had never seen one before. As I was doing treatments, I noticed a dog needed 2.2cc of enrofloxacin (an antibiotic). For some reason, I read 22cc. I always taught nurses that if you give a small animal 22cc of anything, you are probably wrong, and if you give a 200 pound Great Dane .2cc of anything, again, you are most likely mistaken. But I did not heed my own advice as I drew up 22cc of the drug and proceeded to inject the small terrier mix with the entire syringe. I did not realize what I had done until an hour or so later when the owners came in and euthanized the dog. The effects of my mistake would never be seen.

Later that night, a dog came in who had eaten snail bait. The standard treatment is to give the dog apomorphine, a morphine derivative that induces vomiting. The doctor told me the dose, and I did my calculations.

I gave the dog the injection, and he started to vomit so violently he could not stop. It took more than an hour for him to stop vomiting when it should have only taken about 10 minutes. The doctor asked me if I gave the dose she asked for. Through talking with her, I realized I had given ten times the dose!

In a weird sort of way, I think I did the dog a service, because the snail bait came up after he had been vomiting for about forty-five minutes. The prescribed dose would not have done the job.

It was pure luck that both of the cases turned out all right. But it does not change the fact that I could have killed both patients. I talked to my supervisor, after the apomorphine incident, and she sent me home. I got into bed that night and cried. I cried not only because of the mistakes I had made, but because I was looking forward to an indefinite period of time in bed.

I finally cried for all I had lost. But most of all, I cried because my passion for life was fading. I had to quit my job — my biggest passion in life. This would be the first time I was really sick and bed-ridden. I was terrified, devastated, and did not know what to expect. I slept the best I could that night, and knew my parents were on their way to help me in the morning.

I woke up the next morning and got dressed. The doorbell rang shortly after, and when I answered the door, my parents audibly gasped. My face was hollow, and my eyes sunken. I had also put on more weight — and they could not believe the difference in the few weeks since they had seen me last.

After they hugged me, my mom proclaimed, "We're taking you home."

My first thought was complete and total relief. I was being rescued. The second, my job, and what I was going to tell them. We decided to go to lunch to talk about what to do next. While at the restaurant, my mom gave me a necklace. It was

"Footprints in the Sand". On the front was an abstract beach with footprints on it, and on the back it read "It was during those times that I carried you."

I cried, and realized I was not alone.

My parents wanted me to come home with them that day. When I got back to my house after lunch, I called work, and spoke to the office manager. I explained to him I would not be back, and I was sorry I could not give notice.

He exclaimed, "Well that's just great, I hope you never plan to work here again!" He quickly hung-up the phone on me.

My initial reaction was horror and embarrassment. But I decided not to let it get to me. I had other things to worry about.

Next, I talked to my landlord and explained my situation. I told her I would pay the next month's rent since I could not give her thirty days' notice. This way, I could move out slowly. She was so kind and understanding and appreciated the financial gesture. However, she explained, it was not necessary. I gave her the money anyway.

My parents and I packed as much as we could in the car, and I drove home that day with them. Nothing compared to that first night at home. I did not have to worry about getting up and going to work, I did not have to worry about money, and I did not have to worry about being alone. I slept really well that night, but I woke up every day feeling worse.

We rented a U-Haul about a week later, and my parents and brother went down to San Diego once again to move everything home. I helped as much as I could, but mainly, I just told them what belonged to me.

Most of my stuff ended up in storage, but my parents were able to make the loft (outside of my bedroom) into a small living room. It was like a little apartment. This way, I did not have to go up and down the stairs and I could have some privacy. They did everything in their power to make my life as simple and easy as possible.

Shortly after I moved home, Jennifer found out I was not feeling well and drove more than an hour to surprise me and tell me that she loved me.

It hurt me that I was too sick to go to lunch and spend time catching up that day, but she said, "It's all right, Steph, I'll just sit with you and if you need to sleep, go right ahead and if you want to talk — I'm here."

And she did just that. She did not expect me to talk or hang out. She just sat with me! I knew right then she would always be one of my best friends.

I will forever love her for that.

This was the first time I became so sick that I could not work or function. It was about four months before I could get up and start to live a semi-functional life. I am so fortunate I had my family to fall back on. Otherwise, I would have fought this alone, and I do not think I would have made it through.

Even with a great family, it is still a very lonely fight. And even though I recovered in four months, each time I have gotten sick, it has lasted longer and longer. And as of yet, I have seen no end in sight.

Health Clinics

*T*found an intensive health clinic through my mom. She worked at my high school alma mater, and had received a call from a woman named Susan, regarding her daughter. The woman explained how her daughter had Chronic Fatigue Syndrome, and had been unable to attend school for many years.

Susan suffered from CFIDS as well.

Her daughter was extremely sick and, in fact, had developed bedsores from lying in bed so long. Sadly, she had been experiencing fatigue problems from the time she was five years old. She had been in and out of school during the last six or seven years. Her childhood had been stolen from her. All she wanted was to be a normal teenager.

Susan hired a home-school teacher and tutors to try to keep her up to date with the other students, but now, Susan said her daughter was starting to feel better — and was hoping she could start attending school on a part time basis.

My mom talked to her, in depth, about her daughter's illness and explained that her own daughter had also been recently diagnosed with CFIDS. Susan said when she gave birth to her daughter, she was quite sick with the illness.

The only way for her to take care of her new infant daughter was to keep her in the bed next to her. She fed her, changed her, and maintained all of her interactions with the new baby from her bed. She believed it was possible she transmitted the disease either while she was pregnant or during her daughter's infancy.

Susan and her husband had divorced by the time the baby was five. Her daughter would go and stay with her father and when she complained to him about being tired, he felt she was being lazy. After all, he thought, she was a kid, and they all need some tough love.

In her early teens, her dad would fill a backpack with rocks and force her to, not only wear it, but run up and down stadium stairs in an effort to make her stop being so lazy. Susan also explained she was starting to see signs of CFIDS in her second daughter who was, at the time, eight years old.

Susan attributed a renowned health clinic for saving her daughter's life. They had not cured her daughter or completely alleviated the problem, but they had been able to get her to a functional state. The doctors were compassionate and took her complaints seriously. They had given her supplements, IV fluid infusions, and changed her diet. This helped her daughter enough that she wanted to start attending school. She wanted to be a normal teenager.

I think for the first time, my mom was able to hear a story from another sufferer, and she was deeply affected by Susan's life. I think she was able to see how real and destructive CFIDS was.

I never doubted for a second my family believed me, but it rekindled their belief that we could do something about it. We did not have to just sit by and watch as CFIDS ruined my life — as well as the lives of those around me. Finally, we would be given an opportunity to feel like we were fighting — to take an active and proactive role in my health. For the previous couple of years, since my diagnosis, we had felt completely help-less. There were no resources available to help me cope, or help my family fight.

I still wanted the "magic bullet" that would cure the CFIDS. I just wanted to have a pill that would make it go away. I was so desperate I was willing to try anything. I would easily commit to any drug or treatment a doctor suggested. I did not care about side effects or long-term damage; I needed something to allow me to function every day — and I needed it now.

My mom and I went to the health clinic to gain as much information as we could. They offered a comprehensive health "week". This involved staying at a local hotel and attending seminars, learning how to eat properly, and having a battery of tests run to determine what — if anything — was wrong.

People flew in from all over the country to attend this life-changing week.

This clinic was a last resort for many people after being told by their doctors they had two months to live. They suffered from diseases like cancer and heart disease. Surprisingly, many of the people, after making the appropriate dietary and exercise changes were still alive many years later.

The health clinic was now starting to address immune-mediated diseases such as CFIDS and fibromyalgia. Unfortunately, they had a long way to go in this field, but the fact that they addressed the issues and problems associated with the diseases was a huge step in the right direction.

My sales counselor was the mother, Susan, from the earlier story. We talked for a long time about the program, how it has changed other people's lives, and how it would benefit me.

She suggested that even though I lived close by, I should stay in the hotel with the rest of the participants. The days were long and demanding, and she thought it would be helpful if I had a place to lie down during the day, and did not have to make the drive to and from the clinic in traffic. She understood how important it was for CFIDS patients to rest throughout the seminar.

Without the hotel room, there was nowhere for me to sleep. I decided I wanted to try an intensive treatment option and was excited to start the program. I could not wait to start the IV infusions that had helped Susan's daughter so dramatically. I clung to the hope they would work for me.

The estimated price of the week was $10,000. At the time, I was not working and unable to obtain independent health insurance, and I went into sticker shock. My parents, amazing as they are, did not blink an eye. If it would help, they would do whatever was necessary to "fix" their daughter. They were not wealthy people, and they would have sold their house and every possession they had if need be. But, at twenty-six years old, I still felt terrible that I was still relying on them for money.

I just was not in a position to fend for myself. I was on government disability, unable to work and living at home. My life had been turned upside down, and again, I had to ask my parents for help. We decided to register for the first available opening and my mom wrote the check for the deposit.

The demand for the comprehensive week of treatment was extremely high, and it was difficult to find a spot for me. It was also important for me to see one particular doctor who had spent a great deal of time working with CFIDS patients. With a little bit of creative scheduling, Susan was able to get me into the following week's seminars.

The program began on Sunday evening. My parents wanted to go with me to check into the hotel, and sign up for the seminars. Everything but the medical testing took place in the hotel, and they provided a shuttle to the clinic so I did not need my own car. I entered a medium-sized conference room on the first floor of the hotel and walked over to the tables set up along the perimeter.

I signed in and my mom gave them the "balance owed" check. I grabbed a few munchies provided for attendees, but the food offered was not very appealing. A whole-wheat pita filled with sprouts and a tomato, a piece of fruit, and a cup of herbal tea. From there, I was given the key to my room, and my parents and I went upstairs to settle in.

I looked over the paperwork they gave me and was horrified by the menu. There was nothing on it I would ever — not in a million years — eat. I tried to look on the bright side though; maybe I would lose some weight.

The seminars during the week included: preventing heart disease, prostate cancer, diabetes, high blood pressure, hormone therapy, menopause, and angina. None of these topics applied to me, and I was a little disappointed.

Susan had warned me, though, the week focused on older people, and the issues they face. She said I would probably be the youngest person there. And I was — by thirty or more years.

I knew I would be sleeping most of the day, and I was hoping to have IV infusions all week, so I quickly dismissed the idea that the seminars were not relevant to my condition. I immediately decided that I would not feel bad for missing the classes, after all, I was really sick. I planned on attending the things that were important or interesting to me, and then I'd sleep the rest of the time.

The first day was the hardest. At seven o'clock in the morning, I went to a nurse's station, which was in one of the hotel rooms on the second floor. They took my vitals, weight, and blood pressure. Then they gave me a vitamin B complex shot. From there I went to the same conference room I checked in at the night before.

The room now had large, round tables that seated ten and they were filled with people eating breakfast. But the food was never very appealing. Everything was whole and pure, and a little strange, I might add. I wanted the processed food and the sugar, and I left that morning quite hungry.

After breakfast, I was shuttled to the clinic for my prelimi-
nary meeting with the doctor. The appointment was about two
hours long, and my mom had come to sit in. The doctor
spent the first hour getting my detailed history. She wrote
down everything I said. Then she explained her thoughts and
feelings regarding CFIDS and various theories she believed
contributed to the syndrome.

She was one of the few people, outside of my family, who
told me she believed me. For the first time, I felt respected,
and justified. She ordered every blood panel under the sun.
Food allergies, vitamin levels, heavy metals screening, organ
functions, CBC, urinalysis, candida levels, adrenal gland
function — you name it, she ran it. Her nurse took at least
twenty vials of blood.

After my blood was taken, the doctor started me on some
basic natural vitamins. When my test results returned and she
had a chance to analyze them, she said there would be more
supplements added to the regimen. I asked about the IV infusions, and she decided to start them immediately. The first
one would be after lunch. I was so sick, and I was hoping for
immediate results. I could not wait!

When my appointment was over, I got on the shuttle and
went back to the hotel for lunch. My mom went to a local fast
food restaurant with the agreement we would meet back at the
clinic for my first infusion drip.

The meals were very rigidly scheduled, and if you missed
one, you had to make other arrangements. Again, the food
was not very appealing. A lot of soy and vegetables — the very
things I worked so hard to avoid. Once again, I left a bit hungry. After lunch, I got back on the shuttle and returned to the
clinic for my first IV fluid drip.

I was led over to a large room that had approximately five
circles of six recliners. I signed in at the desk, was told to

take a seat in one of the recliners, and a nurse would be right with me. My mom sat with me and we waited only a short time before Jean came over. She took my vitals and then prepared to place a catheter. She was very abrupt with me and slightly grumpy, but over the next few months, I grew to love her. I would not let any other nurse place my IV catheters.

I always refused to allow her to put the catheters in my hand, and made her place them in my arm. After putting in the catheter, she explained the infusion was mainly vitamins, and it should take about two hours to have all the liquid drip into my body. She said I might feel a little flush or nauseous, and if I did, they could slow it down. She started the drip and I leaned my head back and tried to relax.

My mom looked at me and started to cry. She said it was so hard to see me sitting there with a tube in my arm. I was so sick and my face had grown hollow. The dark circles around my eyes had become deep black pits. When I leaned my head back and the light was just right, my face looked like a skeleton. It broke her heart. She prayed these infusions would help. She felt so defenseless. To watch her child suffer with no relief in sight was unbearable for her.

It did not take long for the IV fluid to pass through my system. I would get up every ten minutes or so to use the restroom. Because of this, I was not able to sleep during the infusion time, so I was always completely exhausted when the drip was finished. After the drip was done, my mom went home, and I went back to the hotel.

By this time, dinner was being served, and I walked into the conference room and sat at my usual table. I made some very small talk with those at my table, and over the week grew to appreciate the camaraderie between us. I really only saw them at meals because I was too exhausted to attend the classes, but they were all very supportive and understanding.

Once again, I picked at my food. I was starting to get hungry enough I ate some of the things I would not normally and found things were starting to taste okay. After dinner, I decided to attend the one seminar that looked appealing.

We entered another conference room filled with chairs and I took my seat when suddenly, a guy burst into the room dressed in a Hawaiian shirt, jeans, and sandals. His hair resembled a mad scientist and he had the most cheerful face I had seen in a long time. He exuded excitement and oozed of compassion. From the moment he opened his mouth I adored him. I guessed him to be in his late forties or early fifties and he was a chiropractor who worked at the clinic. He said the clinic patients benefited greatly from being treated by him during the week they spent attending the seminar.

He was different than any chiropractor I was used to. He did not believe in coming in to be adjusted unless you had a reason. He said that years ago, when he was a new chiropractor, he was seeing this woman a number of times a week. He had not needed to adjust her during her last few visits, and started to feel guilty for charging his fee without actually doing anything but examine her. So he decided that during her next visit, he would adjust her whether she needed it or not.

The patient came in and, again, the chiropractor realized that she was fine, but decided to go ahead with the adjustment. She paid her bill and left. A few hours later, she called him to report that a severe migraine had developed after she left the office. He had her return, and he claimed it took him almost one week of daily adjustments to completely alleviate the migraine he caused.

From that day on, he only adjusted his patients when they needed it. He also believed patients should only need to be adjusted a few times for a given problem. If a chiropractor has a patient coming in for a year or more for the same problem, he is not doing his job right. He would give his clients an idea of how long he would need to treat them so they were not constantly coming in without an end in sight.

Most of his cases were resolved in only three to five visits.

His lecture lasted for about two hours, and he was so funny and informative I was actually disappointed when it was over. I caught myself belly laughing for the first time in as long as I could remember. During the seminar, he had his massage therapists walking around giving mini-massages to everyone who attended.

He ended by suggesting we should all consider seeing him for an evaluation, and having a massage by one of his therapists. They sat in the back of the room and made appointments for those of us who were interested. I booked a massage for the next day — and right after, would see the chiropractor.

I dragged myself upstairs and collapsed into bed. I called my parents and explained the rest of my day. My mom suggested I get a massage every day, but I decided I did not want to commit to that much time, so I planned to have two that week. I was feeling so drained already, and this was only the first day. If this was any indication of the pace I could anticipate, I did not think I would make it through the rest of the week.

From then on, I made my schedule fairly simple. I would wake in the morning at seven. This was really difficult for me, but I kept reminding myself it was only for one week. I would have my vitals taken, receive my vitamin B shot, eat breakfast, get my drip, have lunch, get some sleep, have dinner, and then retire for the night. On two of the days, I saw the chiropractor and had a massage. But every day after the first, I made sure I was able to sleep for the better part of the day.

On Friday, I was ready to see the doctor again, and get the results to my many, many tests. There were very few findings. My adrenal glands were functioning at peak levels all the time. This did not allow for my body to adjust to stress. By having them constantly on the alert, my body thought it was on the defensive twenty-four hours a day. There was no way for it to rest.

She also found some B vitamin deficiencies and started me on injectable B complex. Every day I was to give myself shots in my hips. This would go on indefinitely for now. But, by far, the most interesting finding of all was my food allergy panel. It tested for all sorts of fruits, vegetables, meats, poultry, fish, grains, fats, etc. and it was quite comprehensive. According to the test, the only things I was not allergic to were plums and spinach.

The doctor put me on approximately 25 different supplements.

I was to take some with food, some on an empty stomach.

Take some with water, some without.

Take this one alone.

Take this one with that one.

This one is three times a day.

That pill is four times a day.

The other one is five times a day.

I had detailed written instructions on how to take all of my new pills. When all was said and done, I was taking about seventy-five to one hundred pills a day. She also had me stop the Prozac as well as the birth control pill on the following cycle.

After seeing the doctor, I went straight to the nutritionist so she could help me put together a meal plan that would best suit my health problems. The nutritionist sat for some time staring at the food allergy panel. Finally, she put down the test, looked me square in the eye, and said, "I'm sorry, but I don't know what to tell you to eat."

Her frustration was evident, and her confusion by the results was obvious. She said she had never seen a test that looked like this.

She thought about it some more and commented there were other grains not listed on the test I might be able to try.

Unfortunately, I was so allergic to all of the tested grains that I would probably find the same to be true of the alternatives. However, she felt it might be worth a try. She suggested things such as quinoa, spelt, and various other grains that could only be found in health food stores.

There were cookbooks I could buy that would teach me how to make my own breads with these grains and use them in various recipes. But the problem was, all the recipes required eggs, soy, milk, or rice and, according to my test results, I could not eat any of these things.

After health week was over, my mom and I went to the health food store and scoured the shelves for anything I could eat. It was really slim pickings. Everything contained many of the very things I was so allergic to. We found and bought a few cookbooks for allergies and bought seven or eight different flours to start experimenting at home.

What a miserable failure that was. The food tasted terrible, and I had to do so many substitutions that nothing even looked as it should. Between the vitamin regimen and trying to find things to eat, I was busy all day long. Within a few weeks, I was so exhausted and frustrated I just about collapsed.

I decided to try to eat reasonably well, even if I did eat my allergic foods. I faithfully continued the vitamins and other pills, went off of Prozac and the birth control pill, and kept a close eye on my diet.

I continued to be checked by the doctor from the health week and would have an occasional adjustment and massage with the chiropractor. Overall, I continued to sleep for eighteen to twenty hours a day and just tried to maintain a low-stress lifestyle.

Within a short time after stopping the Prozac, my hip and shoulder joints began to hurt. The chiropractor took a few x-rays of my shoulder, and had a radiologist look at them. He said there was no overt abnormality, and based on my age and history would guess that I had fibromyalgia. A relatively new disease related to CFIDS that was characterized by unexplained joint pain. There was no test, no cure, and no treatment at this point. I was right back in the same position — only now, I had two diseases.

This was a pretty devastating blow after all I had been through. I could not believe what I was hearing. I had also noticed my mood shifting in a downward direction and, after two months, made the hard decision to go back on Prozac. Within a couple of weeks, my mood started to lift and after a month or so, my aches and pains had gone away. My muscles were still tight and tense, but I knew it was a result of being in bed for days at a time.

Soon, the vitamins started to get too expensive, and I questioned whether they were really helping. I had given them four months and did not notice a significant change. I recovered slowly — as I had in the past. After the usual three to four months, I was starting to get back on my feet. Even with all the medical help, my recovery time was the same. After spending $300-400 a month for four months, I decided to stop the vitamins. I was spending so much energy, money, and time keeping up with them throughout the day I was not able to rest, as I should have all along.

Through quite a bit of independent research, I found the food allergy panels could be a reflection of my overall health. The sicker a person is, the more allergic they will appear. My body was in such a compromised state when the test was done that it was no surprise to show such shocking results. After finding this information, I decided to ignore the food allergy panel and continued to eat reasonably healthy.

The doctor I had been seeing finally moved on to another practice, and I started seeing a different doctor at the clinic. I also started to have bad pain in my lower left abdomen, and my periods were off kilter.

The doctor I saw recommended going to an OB/GYN. I asked for a referral and he said his wife saw a doctor in Newport Beach and was very pleased with her.

This, unfortunately, brought to light another huge health issue that had been lingering since I was a young teen. She would find problems I still battle today: ovarian cysts, endometriosis, and breast lumps. I made my appointment with her and hoped she would be able to help me.

Now What's Wrong?

I had no idea what to expect when I went off the birth control pill for the first time in more than twelve years. I was convinced part of my problem could be contributed to being on the hormones for so long. By ridding my body of all of the drugs I was taking, I might find some relief to my symptoms.

The idea made sense, and it sounded right. All those years of fighting my natural body systems and trying to alter nature had, undoubtedly, taken its toll. How could my body know what it is supposed to do when I had never given it the opportunity to function on its own?

In December of 1998, I took my last birth control pill. I was thrilled to be done with it, but was petrified due to my history of mood swings when I was younger.

The last time I was "drug-free" was when I was fifteen years old. What was I to expect? I was not looking forward to becoming an unpredictable nightmare again.

Soon, I realized I was not experiencing the terrible mood swings that had caused me so much difficulty in the past. I was by no means even-keeled every second, but the severe emotional changes I saw as a teenager did not happen.

Unfortunately, though, my face broke out extremely bad, and I looked as if I was going through puberty all over again. The pill had kept my skin flawless over the years, and I had difficulty accepting my "new" face. I was embarrassed by the amount of acne that developed — and I had to start dealing with not only the tremendous exhaustion and previous weight gain, but also the disfiguring pimples.

Oddly enough, during most of this, I was still pretty sick. I did not see the life-changing effects on my health I had hoped to achieve. Most of the time I would dismiss all of the emotional pain because I was fighting to stay awake for longer than an hour at a time. But when I looked in the mirror or went out in public, I was ashamed and humiliated.

In May 1999, I started to have pain in the lower left side of my abdomen. There was pain when I had a bowel movement and when gas passed through my colon. I thought it was my ovary, but I could not be sure. My history would point to a cyst, but this pain was far worse than any I'd experienced before. If it were a cyst, I imagined it was fairly large.

I returned to the health center, and the doctor referred me to Dr. Jones, OB/GYN. I made an appointment for a day or two later to see her nurse practitioner. The appointment desk informed me that Dr. Jones was unable to see new patients for a few months, but because of the pain I was experiencing, they wanted me to come in immediately.

Within a few minutes of seeing the nurse practitioner, she directed me to the ultrasound room. My mom and I sat in the waiting room for a few minutes before they called me in. I'd had many ultrasounds in the past, so I had no reason to believe this one would be any different. I undressed, and got on the table.

The beginning of the study was routine. The technician made a few comments during the test that she saw something that was suspicious. She guessed it was a cyst on the left ovary.

She set the probe down, and wiped off my abdomen.

As I watched her, thinking the test was over, she removed a condom from the drawer and placed it over a very long and slender probe. This time, she explained, she needed to insert this probe into my vagina so should would be able to get a better view of the ovaries. I felt a tremendous amount of pain as she pushed the probe in and moved it around inside of me. But in the end, the doctor was able to get a complete look at my entire pelvic cavity.

When the ultrasound was over, I put my clothes on, walked out of the room and said to my mom, "She found something".

We went back into the exam room and the nurse practitioner returned. She said the radiologist looked over the images — and there was a cyst on my left ovary the size of a plum. She, Dr. Jones, and the radiologist, felt a surgical exploratory would be needed. She briefly explained the procedure — called a laparoscopy — and I scheduled an appointment the next week to have a pre-op consultation with Dr. Jones.

The following week I met with the doctor for the first time and she went over the surgery in detail. I would have three small holes punctured into my abdomen. One through the navel and the other two would be below the pubic hairline. She would then insert instruments so she could look into the abdomen. They would inflate my abdomen with carbon dioxide gas so it would provide more room to look at my internal organs, and also use a laser to drain the cyst.

There was a small chance the ovary would have to be removed and an even smaller chance I would have to be cut open for traditional surgery. The only way to know was after she had gotten a look inside. She also said there was a possibility I had endometriosis — when the uterine tissue is found outside the uterus — but she would laser it off if she found any.

The surgery was scheduled for a few days after our consultation. I had my pre-op blood work done and went home to wait. The morning of the surgery came, and I was petrified. I'd had surgery on my knee about five years before and I woke up extremely nauseous, agitated, confused, and I could not urinate.

I hated the "waking up" part. I fought it as hard as I could, and it was a very scary experience. This time, I wanted my rosary in the room with me. I felt it would be able to offer me some of the support I had lacked, years prior, during my knee surgery.

The nurse assured me that the small wood beads would be by my head during the procedure and she would let the anesthesiologist know I wanted it in the room. That little string of beads gave me so much comfort and I knew it would guide my surgeon to do the best job possible.

I explained my terror to my anesthesiologist the morning of the operation and he was reassuring. He really put me at ease. He put in the IV catheter, and gave me an injection of Versed — a drug given to surgery patients because it not only relaxes you, but it causes some level of amnesia.

The idea is you should not remember being wheeled into the operating room, getting onto the table, and being given the gas. I told myself I was going to pay attention. I worked in the operating room with animals after all, and I wanted to see their set-up, the equipment they use, and the all-around way they ran a human surgery suite.

All I remember is saying, "I help with surgery on animals."

I do not remember the gas mask, the injection, getting on the table, the staff, or the room. All I remember is that one line!

Before I knew it, the recovery nurse was saying, "Stephanie, open your eyes! Surgery is done! You are in recovery! Everything is fine!"

I said, in slurred speech, "Is Dr. Jones going to tell me what she found?"

The nurse chuckled and said, "Honey, she already told you,

and is back at the office seeing appointments. She talked to your parents and they will tell you what she said."

She told me to rest and close my eyes. I noticed a clock on the wall, and tried to note the time. I also tried to move my hands, and realized I had my rosary clutched in them. Again, that simple string of beads made everything all right.

The next thing I knew, I opened my eyes and about an hour had passed. Or did I misread the clock the first time? Anyway, the nurse came over and raised the back of the bed a little so I was almost sitting up. I asked if she would bring in my parents. She did, and it was so wonderful to see them.

They hugged and kissed me, and my mom had a little cry. They said the cyst was quite large, and Dr. Jones removed it without damaging my ovary. I also had a moderate amount of endometriosis she burned off with the laser. She did a complete exam of my uterus and fallopian tubes and felt I should have no problems having children one day.

We did not know anything about endometriosis, but she would explain it further at my post-op appointment two days later. She had said, though, I should feel tremendously better, and felt the surgery was very productive.

I continued to wake up and the nurses started to encourage me to use the bathroom. The procedure was outpatient and therefore, I had to urinate before going home.

I got up and went into the bathroom. I had to go, but I could not. I went back and forth from bed to restroom for about two hours, and was not able to pass a drop. The nurses had me try everything, but nothing worked. I soon had to go so bad, I was experiencing a tremendous amount pain — it felt like my bladder would rupture any minute. The nurses called Dr. Jones, and she instructed them to catheterize me.

I cannot describe the incredible feeling when that catheter passed into my bladder and it started to empty. The pain was instantly gone. For some reason, I was able to urinate thirty minutes after they removed the catheter.

A silent cheer rang through the entire recovery room as I came out of the bathroom, punched my fist into the air and said, "I went!" It had been a grueling four hours.

I was discharged with my post-op instructions, and sent on my way. When I got home, I slept for a little while that afternoon, but the pain was so minimal I was up and making a sandwich for dinner that night. My parents, of course, wanted to "nurse" me, but I felt all right. I did not feel much pain, and it felt good to be up and moving a little.

I would get tired very quickly. This limited my activity and I found I was on my back a lot. My parents tried to explain that the pain medication they gave me had probably not worn off yet, and I should take it really easy. After all, I was only a few hours out of abdominal surgery. But, of course, what did they know — I felt pretty darn good!

The next morning, I woke up and felt like a truck had run me over! The pain was not severe; I was just extremely sore. The leftover carbon dioxide gas they used to inflate my abdomen had traveled into my shoulder joints and chest cavity. It made my shoulders ache, and caused me to be short of breath.

There was still some excess gas that remained in my abdomen and every time I rolled over, I could feel my organs move around as the gas fought its way to the highest point.

The incisions themselves just felt like deep cuts, so there was mild discomfort at the penetration sites, but all around them was very tender. I was also bleeding like I was having a light period (which is normal for a laparoscopy), so I was fighting with sanitary pads — no tampons allowed.

Within two or three days, I was really up and moving. I went to my post-op appointment where Dr. Jones removed the stitches and explained what she found. Again, she had removed the cyst and lasered off the endometriosis.

Dr. Jones found more endometriosis than she had anticipated, and said it would definitely explain why I felt so bad. She showed me pictures and insisted I go back on the pill. In addition, she felt I should suppress my periods for three months at a time so it would slow down the build-up of the endometriosis.

After I started feeling better, I started to do some research on endometriosis, and found it is not only misunderstood, but can only be diagnosed through a laparoscopy. Most people think, incorrectly, that endometriosis is a thickening of the lining of the uterus.

In actuality, the theory behind the condition is during your period, the blood and sloughed uterine tissue backs up and exits out of the fallopian tubes instead of leaving the body through the vagina. From there, these tiny pieces of tissue attach to the organs in the abdomen.

Every month, the tissue responds like uterine tissue and starts to swell. At the time of menstruation, the tissue in the abdomen starts to bleed as well. This causes a build up of free blood in the abdominal cavity every month. Not only is this painful, but it takes the body awhile to absorb the excess blood, and then the cycle starts all over again.

The basic theory is if menstruation is suppressed, there is no bleeding — and therefore, less chance of the tissue build up throughout the abdomen. Also, the pill can cause periods to be lighter and shorter, and this aids in reducing the reoccurrence of the endometriosis.

There are many theories related to this phenomenon, but no one has been able to figure out exactly why it happens. The fact is the tissue has been found throughout the body, including the lymph system, and the brain. It can block the fallopian tubes and cause infertility; while at the same time can strangle the bladder, intestine, or bowels.

It can cause such damage the only "cure" is a complete hysterectomy. There is no explanation, but doctors have found that pregnancy seems to dramatically reduce the occurrence of build up.

Because of this, Dr. Jones asked, "Are you planning to get pregnant anytime soon?"

After controlling my laughter I explained that I did not even have a dating prospect, and would probably wait for a little while.

"Well, you might want to make it sooner rather than later," she said.

Within about two weeks, I started feeling like becoming more active. I went out in the back yard and swam a few laps. I was winded quick, but it was different. I was tired because I was exercising, not just trying to get out of bed.

Slowly over the next few weeks, I swam more and more laps. I felt stronger and healthier.

I took SCUBA lessons three months after surgery, and felt better than I had in years. My parents and I determined this was what was wrong with me all along. I never had CFIDS after all! It was endometriosis the whole time.

I started working again, took a few trips, and started to rekindle some friendships.

But by April of 2000, I started to feel that familiar feeling. The fatigue was creeping in again. The desire to plan my sleep and the inability to maintain my personal hygiene started, once again, taking over my life.

I immediately called Dr. Jones, and she saw me right away. She felt there might be a small build-up in the endometriosis, but in a years time, and all the suppressing of my periods we did, she did not feel there would be much there. We could go into surgery again, but she was not sure it was necessary — or we could wait and see what happened.

I went home depressed and defeated. I still felt the endometriosis was my problem. A few days later, I called her back and begged her to do another surgery. I was desperate; I was getting sick again and I needed a quick fix!

Dr. Jones agreed, knowing she could not always get all of the endometriosis the first time. She had warned me after my first surgery that there was a small possibility, within a year, I would need to have it done again. I felt that maybe we would luck out and find more endometriosis.

The second surgery was May 2000, and it went the same way as the first. Again, I was scared to death, but everyone involved helped me stay calm. Dr. Jones did find more endometriosis, but considered it to be mild. She felt it was a worthwhile endeavor, and hoped I would feel better. I went home and waited for the amazing results I'd had the year before.

But those results never came.

My belief I did not have CFIDS started to fade. It crept up behind me and snatched my life once again.

I tried going off the pill again in December 2001 while I was fighting another round of CFIDS. I thought, once again, my troubled health might be fixed without all of the medicinal help. Within six months, I was having a tremendous amount of abdominal bloating and discomfort. I was grouchy all the time, and felt like I always had the flu. I looked like I was six months pregnant most of the time. The CFIDS was starting to resolve, but I could not get over the horrible endometriosis symptoms.

I consulted with Dr. Jones again in July 2002. I was engaged, and my fiancé and I wanted to start a family the following year in March. She offered a few options.

I could go back on the pill, and see how I did. I could have surgery right then, and possibly need another one before we tried to get pregnant. I could hold out and have surgery later so I probably would not need another one before March — or I could just deal with it. Whatever I chose she felt I should go back on the pill and suppress my periods anyway.

I went home, and my fiancé and I talked long and hard about the options. In the end, I could not take the pain and discomfort any more, and I had a third surgery in September 2002. Again, it went much as the first two, but the doctor found a lot of endometriosis on my uterus and ovaries. In fact, she was surprised to see so much build up after only two years.

I went back on the pill, and started to suppress again.

I found that while I had been off of the pill, I rarely got cold sores, and my migraines were somewhat under control. Going back on the pill caused my cold sores to get completely out of control. I would have six or seven at one time, and I rarely had times when I did not have at least one on my lips.

My migraines were fine when I was suppressing, but when I would have a period every three months, I would have four or five migraines during the week I menstruated.

All of these things were a small price to pay. I was worried about fertility issues and if this was what I had to do, then I would do it. It started to not be about me and more about the future life I might bring into the world and my future husband who wanted children so badly.

As of now, the endometriosis is under control. Hopefully, having a baby will rid me of it. The third surgery had good results on my health, but I was not sick with CFIDS when I had the procedure.

I just hope and pray that when I am ready to have children, I will have a normal pregnancy, and healthy babies. My outlook is good, but with my history, I am not so sure. My husband and I talk about it frequently and can only hold a positive thought for our future.

But You Don't Look Depressed

*M*y parents were always healthy and happy and only suffered minor colds and ailments. My mom has always had high blood pressure and over the last ten years or so has suffered from a TIA (small stroke) or two. They are focused in her eye and she loses her peripheral vision when she has one. The doctors have not been too concerned about her because really, there is not a whole lot that can be done. She is on blood pressure medication and takes a mild blood thinner.

My family, on the whole, has been very lucky in the health department. I was the unfortunate one who constantly had problems and was always at the doctor.

But this all changed in September 2000.

My dad had retired from his job in March of that year and both my parents looked forward to retirement in a brand new home in a beautiful community in Palm Desert, California.

They were able to buy a house on the first tee box of the golf course and started to settle into their peaceful new life. For thirty-five years their life took place in Orange County and they spent a good deal of time at my condominium as they started to shift their life out to the desert.

My parents were visiting me one afternoon after I had been fighting with CFIDS for about four months. I was slowly starting to get back on my feet by working a day or two a week and spending the rest of the time resting and sleeping. On this particular day I had gone upstairs to take a nap after we had gone to breakfast and run a few errands. My parents, too, were tired and both laid down on the couches downstairs.

I was just starting to fall asleep when my mom came into my room. I sleepily looked at her.

"Your father is having chest pains, I think we need to take him to the hospital," she whispered.

The drowsiness that lingered in my head immediately vanished and I jumped out of bed.

"We should take him to Hoag Hospital," my mom explained.

My mind processed the information as quickly as possible and I knew we needed to go to the emergency room that was only one block away. Even though Hoag Hospital was one of the top hospitals in the area, it would take twenty to thirty minutes to get there, and who knew what the traffic would be like. Time was of the essence at the moment.

I threw on sweats and a sweatshirt and ran downstairs.

My dad was lying on the couch, holding his chest, and breathing extremely shallow and fast. We carefully led him to the car and helped him sit down.

We arrived at the emergency room in five minutes. I ran in, ahead of my dad, and told the receptionist I thought my dad was having a heart attack.

By the time he got to the door with my mom, there was a wheelchair and orderly waiting for him. They immediately took him in the back and started working on him. My mom and I were not allowed to go with him initially but they kept us busy with paperwork.

After ten or fifteen minutes we still had not heard anything so I asked the receptionist if she had any information. She left the front office and immediately returned telling us that he was stable and we could go in the back and see him.

We walked through the door from the waiting room and moved through a series of sterile walkways. We turned the corner and entered the cubicle my dad was being treated in.

I could have never been prepared for what I saw.

He was in a hospital gown, had an IV catheter in his hand, and was a sickly gray color. I had never seen either of my parents sick, they always cared for me — and for the first time, the roles were reversed. I was always the one having the surgeries, seeing endless doctors, and being stuck by all the needles — not my dad. I never had to play the helpless bystander watching and praying everything would be all right.

My dad explained that they had given him a nitroglycerine tablet under his tongue as they were wheeling him into the back room, but there was no effect on his pain. This led them to believe his heart was not the culprit.

That was fantastic news!

They had already taken chest x-rays by the time we were allowed to see him and we were now waiting for the results. We talked about the pain and when and where it started. We were looking for anything he could remember over the last week or two that might have contributed to the situation he was now facing.

Hindsight is twenty-twenty, and every minor symptom he had seemed to have some sort of meaning. He had been tired for a few days, and was having a lot of headaches for the last month or so. Various little remembrances that, previously, had all but been forgotten became extremely important. I tried to understand fully what he was feeling.

The emergency doctor finally came in, and said that his heart looked fine — but he was concerned about his lungs. He suspected bi-lateral pneumonia.

The radiologist told the emergency room doctor to give him a shot for the pain and send him home, but the ER doctor insisted that something was wrong. His gut instinct would not take the radiologist's opinion at face value. He decided to call Dr. Smith, who was a boarded pulmonary specialist. He was also boarded in emergency and critical care medicine, in addition to internal medicine.

The minute Dr. Smith looked at the films and examined my dad, he insisted he be hospitalized, and was amazed he was walking around.

All he kept saying was, "This is a very sick man!"

Over the next few days my dad was on intense IV antibiotics and close observation. Fortunately, he recovered with no complications and was released from the hospital within a few days. It took him about six months to get back on his feet and feel like himself.

I was so impressed with Dr. Smith, and because he was an internal medicine specialist, I decided to see him myself. I made an appointment at the same time my dad had his recheck and we all went to the office.

I was put into an exam room, and had my vitals taken. I sat and waited while my dad had a recheck of his pneumonia. My mom sat in on the recheck with my dad, and then came into the room I was in for my exam.

Dr. Smith came into the exam room and sat down. I went through my whole history again and told him the same things I had explained to every other doctor.

But he seemed different; he really listened.

When I finished my sob story, he started asking questions of his own.

"How many hours do you sleep a day?" he questioned.

"Fourteen to eighteen, but about twelve during the night." I said, and looked at the floor embarrassed. His compassionate manner urged me to continue.

"Do you wake up during the night?" He was writing copious notes.

"Yeah, I go to the bathroom a lot," I replied.

"Really? How often?" the doctor asked.

"Every hour or two." Again, I was embarrassed.

The information obviously registered in his mind, and he continued.

"Are you depressed? " he asked, quite bluntly.

"No," I answered with assurance.

"Do you cry?" he questioned.

I laughed, and said, "No, of course not, I'm on Prozac."

He did not laugh and asked again, "I said, 'Do you cry?'"

It suddenly all came out, I cried for the first time in a long time. I sobbed actually. I wept for all I had lost. The waves of sadness rushed over me, and I almost could not control the tears. The next question hurt the most.

"Do you have any friends?" he asked.

I shook my head "No." I was unable to speak through the tears.

He compassionately asked, "Why?"

"Because I never feel well enough to keep friends." I continued to cry and noticed my mom wipe the tears from her eyes. I cannot imagine the pain she was feeling at this moment, watching her daughter break down.

Dr. Smith stood up, did a thorough exam and said, "I don't know what's wrong with you, but I'm going to do everything I can to find out. I'm not making any promises, but I want to start with a full blood panel. Second, I'm going to give you something to help you sleep. We'll start you on Elavil. You'll take one at night. It's not a sleeping pill, but when you are ready to go to sleep, it will help you sleep deeper."

I left the office with a newfound hope, something I had not felt in years. I immediately went to the pharmacy and had the prescription filled. My parents decided to stay a few more nights since I was starting a new medication. They did not want me to be alone.

The next morning, I came downstairs and both my parents excitedly asked in unison, "Well, how do you feel?"

"Okay, no different, but it has only been one night."

They chuckled at themselves and admitted that it was too early to tell.

Later that day, I felt the same as I had all along and ended up taking a three-hour nap.

Discouraged, I went to bed that night with no expectations.

The next morning, I realized that for the first time, I slept through the night. I did not wake up to go to the bathroom, and I had a full nine hours of uninterrupted sleep. I went downstairs and told my parents. They were thrilled.

We went to breakfast, and throughout the day I slowly started to realize that I was feeling pretty good. My mom and dad wanted to go out and asked if I wanted to tag along.

Normally, I would have been ready to go back to bed, but I surprised myself when I answered, "Yeah, I think I'll go with you."

Every night I slept a little better and every day I felt a little stronger. My life was getting back on track, and I was starting to pick up some hours at work.

I went back to Dr. Smith for my recheck and he could not believe I was the same person. I was smiling and laughing and energized. My blood work had been normal, and he decided to take me off of the Prozac. "Why are you on it anyway?" he questioned.

I explained the story, "I was put on it four years ago so I wouldn't become depressed through all of my health problems and, even worse, I've gained 100 pounds."

"But you don't look depressed." He laughed.

"I know, I've been saying that for years, but everyone keeps telling me that I am."

Once again, I left his office hopeful. Over the next month I slowly went off the Prozac, but continued to take the Elavil. Within two months, I lost twenty-five pounds without effort and I was feeling better than I ever had in my entire life. I was working and living again. I went on a few vacations, and was actively SCUBA diving. My activity level was at an all-time high.

I thought I was cured. I finally found out what was wrong, I was not sleeping well. It was not CFIDS after all.

I put all my focus on getting quality sleep. I did everything in my power to eliminate any and all distractions that might wake or rouse me during the night. I got darker curtains, and did not allow my cats to be in the room when I slept. I removed the phone from my room and started wearing earplugs. Friends and family knew not to call late, and never expected me to answer a phone call after nine each evening.

All of these things worked beautifully for a while. My life was wonderful, full, and active.

But, unbeknownst to me, the clock was ticking and I was about to begin my next round with CFIDS.

Alternative Cures

*O*ver the years my desperation for a cure, or even some sort of treatment, became so intense I would literally try anything. Every ad or article I saw that had a panacea for CFIDS was worth trying. They all claimed that, "Eighty or ninety percent of CFIDS sufferers found a tremendous amount of relief from our product!"

Therefore, needing to believe in something, I tried everything. I bought various pills and tonics, started proclaimed exercise rituals and radical diets. But the end result was always the same; no difference in how I felt. As year after year went by, I wanted to believe that I was taking control of my own health — but I found I would get more and more frustrated after each failed attempt.

Early on in my illness I had decided to try a holistic doctor who my friend had recommended. I went to a number of appointments with no relief in sight.

Not only was it getting quite expensive, but I also had to drive more than a hundred miles to get to him. The experience itself was becoming draining and exhausting. The doctor was unwilling to recommend someone in my area so I decided to stop my appointments altogether. As with every other time I have been sick, rest was what I needed. Within a few months, I was back on my feet and functioning fairly normal.

I have to say, though, that the most interesting thing I have done, "in the name of healing," was to see a healer. She was a referral from a friend of mine who claimed her allergies were eradicated by the unorthodox treatments. She was an hour and a half from my house, and the drive to and from appointments was going to be grueling, but I was excited by the prospect that she might be able to help.

After all, my friend had tremendous results in curing her allergies.

I arrived at her office for my first appointment. We would focus on my history and symptoms. I had already done a few tests with my urine and saliva the prior week and I hoped she would have the results to review with me.

I arrived for my appointment, and when she opened the door, I was a little surprised by her appearance. She was tall and extremely thin. Her tank top and shorts hung on her emaciated frame. Her hair was flaming red and she had the skin texture of leather. It was obvious she had spent far too long in the sun. In fact, I think it was a tanning bed or a self-tanner because she had that orange glow about her. Despite her appearance, her smile was warm and welcoming — and I felt at ease and comfortable with her immediately.

I was led into a small room with a desk and computer along the far wall. She pointed to a couch and asked me to sit down. Directly in front of the sofa was a small office chair where she sat. She spent an hour or two delving deep into my health history, and she worked very hard to understand, fully, what I had been through.

She went over my test results and found that my liver and spleen were compromised. It was important to remember, she explained, that traditional medical testing would not pick up on these imbalances. Testing saliva was far better than any blood test. These tests could pick up on weaknesses in certain organs. It was not to say there was damage or malfunction, just weakness.

After the healer took a thorough history, she led me into a second room that was off the first. It was not lit, yet the light from the outside penetrated the blinds on the windows. All around the room were posters of the various reflexology points, schakra locations, massage techniques, and organ regeneration times. In the center of the room was a massage table with a sheet covering it.

She had me sit on the table. She opened the closet on the opposite wall. Inside was lined with shelves. Each shelf had hundreds of little bottles of pills, tonics, potions, and lotions. She by-passed all of the shelves, and removed two gray brief-cases from the floor.

She returned to the table and opened both of them beside me. Inside were hundreds of small vials, like those perfume samples might come in, and each vial had a small amount of clear liquid in it. The vials were labeled to identify their con-tents. Each vial was organized into a grouping; vitamins, fruits, vegetables, meats, amino acids, various chemicals, fish, grasses, flowers, etc. Within each group were fifteen to twen-ty vials. For example, the fruit category might then be broken down into apples, oranges, bananas, etc. Additionally, each grouping had a combination concoction holding a little of everything in its group.

These little vials, she explained, were going to help us to determine whether or not I was allergic to the essence con-tained within. Her theory was that everything on the face of the planet emits energy. If I am allergic to apples, then hold-ing the apple vial should cause me to lose strength in my body. In a nutshell, the offending substance will drain and sap my energy.

The idea was a little far-fetched to me, but I was open, and willing to try. I held my left arm straight out from my body, parallel to the ground. She pushed down on it as I tried to resist. This was my baseline. She started with the very basics — amino acids and vitamins.

She handed me the vial of amino acids, and I held it in my right hand. I extended my left arm straight out in front of me as she pushed on it. Surprisingly, I found that I had no strength to resist her push. My arm fell to my side with the slightest effort on her part. Next, she did the same thing with each vitamin. Again, my arm fell to my side. It was not surprising to her, considering I was allergic to amino acids and vitamins, that I did not feel well.

Amino acids and vitamins are the building blocks for which all foods are based. My personal belief at the time was that she was pushing harder on my arm at certain times, but again, I was remaining open to the process.

We continued like this for about a half an hour and found that I was affected by almost every category of food. At this point, we did not worry about environmental things like grass and flowers. She was amazed I was so allergic, and it took her a while to determine her plan of attack. She believed she could cure the allergies and, hence, alleviate my health problems. In her eyes, everything was affected by allergies.

What an amazingly simplistic view of the world, I wish it was that easy. I started to buy into it.

The healer decided that because I showed sensitivities to so many things, the best way for us to start was with a fast. It would last for three days and the only things I could ingest were water and elderberry juice (a sweet, dark berry). There were a number of supplements she wanted me to take, in addition to the fast, that would strengthen and detoxify my liver while cleansing the rest of my organs.

It was important to start my treatment immediately, but she could only treat one "allergy" per twenty-four hours, and I had twenty or thirty needing to be addressed. This meant I would need approximately thirty treatments, assuming each treatment was effective the first time. There was occasion she told me when a treatment might need to be repeated.

Even more difficult, after she treated me for an allergy, I was unable to touch, eat, drink, smell, or be exposed to the allergen for at least twenty-four hours. It takes that long for the body to assimilate the new information. By exposing myself to the allergen, I could ruin the work that was done and therefore, need to repeat the previous treatment.

The first treatment was for amino acids and then each vitamin in a very specific order based on how the body broke them down. It was like building a house. You cannot put the roof on without the walls.

I rolled over onto my stomach and she put the amino acid vial in my hand. The next thing I knew, there is this jackhammer-like piece of equipment pounding on my back. She said that, while I was holding the offending allergen, she was opening the various channels throughout my body. This was re-training my system to understand that amino acids were not a threat. The jackhammer pounded on various spots on my neck, back, and the backs of my legs.

At times, it was extremely painful, but I held the belief it was helping.

When the treatment was over, she left the room and let me relax for ten to fifteen minutes because, as she said, it was a fairly traumatic event for the body to go through.

She returned shortly and handed me a piece of paper explaining all of the things I could not touch or eat. Little did I know that amino acids and vitamins were in EVERY-THING, including toothpaste.

I went home, fasted, continued treatments, struggled to stay away from the things that would ruin the current treatment, and commuted back and forth for appointments. Every time I saw her, it was the same thing, only she used a different allergen. And each time, she added more and more supplements. The price was becoming more and more expensive. I was also forbidden to eat most foods and found I was becoming so weak I could hardly stand. I was not feeding my body enough, and I was paying the price for it. I had a constant headache, I was weak, and worst of all, I was constantly dizzy. I was actually feeling worse than before I started treatment, and I think it set my recovery back a month or two.

After about ten treatments over the course of three or four weeks, I mentioned to the healer how much I wanted a piece of pizza or a hamburger. She laughed and expressed her understanding and sympathy, explained I would soon lose those cravings, and said if I did really well and stayed faithful to the regimen I might be able to have a piece of organic chocolate in a year.

I did not think much of the comment, but went home and started to think about the intensity that had developed with this course of treatment. I realized I was not allowing my body to rest. I was so busy avoiding things, commuting, and focusing on my diet, I could not recuperate, as I needed to. In reality I was making myself worse because I was pushing so hard. And, worst of all, I had spent a tremendous amount of money with no end in sight. The bills kept adding up and my credit card kept getting charged.

I made the decision to stop treatment. The weight of the world was off of my shoulders. The healer was not happy about my change in plans, but I did not care. I understood she had invested a lot of time and energy, but I had to do what was right for me.

I started eating again and felt better the next day. I was still very sick, but I was able to stay in bed — what I should have done all along.

Very slowly I recuperated from the stress I inflicted on my body. Who knows if the treatments would have worked, but at the time, I did not have the physical stamina or the financial means to find out.

Sadly, my constant hunt for my magical cure ended there. I was sick of spending thousands of dollars searching and hoping for a cure — only to be left even more tired and tremendously discouraged. CFIDS was my new reality and my best treatment for it was rest and acceptance.

My Knight in Shining Armor

I started to become frustrated with the whole dating scene, and I had resigned myself — at twenty-eight years old — to accept the reality that I might never meet that "special someone".

I had also decided I did not want children. I do not think I believed it, but the odds were stacking up against me. Not only was I getting older with no marital prospects on the horizon, but also I'd had three surgeries for endometriosis already.

My concern was that I might not even be able to conceive a child. And if I did, and carried a child to term, how was I going to take care of an infant when I might get so sick I could barely care for myself.

I did not think I would be able to hold a child in my arms let alone care for it, feed it, and keep it clean. The best way for me to deal with the uncertainty was to avoid it altogether. It was too hard to face the reality of my health, and then try to explain it to the people in my life.

It was easier to have an excuse.

Every grain of my fiber knew I wanted to fall in love and have children, but I wondered how someone could love me with all of my problems.

Over the years, I had dated many different types of men, but the outcome was always the same. My health would deteriorate and I would start to withdraw.

In their defense, I would basically have the attitude that, "This is the way it is, so deal with it!"

Unfortunately, with my attitude, and the doubt most boyfriends felt regarding my disease, it was a recipe for disaster. I curled up in bed, withdrew from life, and they did not understand. It was almost impossible to work through such insurmountable odds.

I was not willing, and they did not care enough to try.

But in January 2001, everything changed, and my life was completely turned upside down. I was completely blind-sided by love.

I was just starting to recover after being sick for a number of months and had recently gone off Prozac when my friend asked if I would be interested in going out on a date with a guy she recently met.

She was using an online dating service to expand her dating pool when a guy named Mike responded to her ad. After one phone call she decided he was too young and she was not interested.

I think she felt sorry for me because I had not been on a date in a while. I was still quite heavy and had been in bed for some time so I think, out of pity, she gave him my number.

Mike called later that night and we talked for six hours! The conversation never lagged for one second and we seemed to "click". We talked about everything.

I did not allow myself to get too excited, but I was looking forward to having someone to hangout with, someone to just go out with and have some fun.

After we had talked for about five hours, I asked if he was interested in what I looked like. He said, "It doesn't matter, I know I like you."

From that moment, I knew I had met someone with compassion and kindness.

Our first phone call was on Wednesday and we set a date for Friday. My parents were in town, so I agreed to meet him at his house. He lived in downtown Huntington Beach, and we planned to walk down to the beach and have dinner at one of the restaurants on the pier. I was nervous because I still weighed 175 pounds and was not at all comfortable with the body I had developed.

I put on an air of confidence, and wore the most flattering clothes I could find. After all, he said he did not care what I looked like, he already liked me. As I pulled up outside his condominium, he was walking out to meet me. He got in the car and helped me find a parking spot. From the moment he sat down, we did not stop talking.

We talked continuously during the walk to the restaurant, during dinner, and the entire walk home. We were like best friends who had not seen each other for a while and were trying desperately to catch up.

When I left that night, I did not know that I was going to fall in love, but I was looking forward to developing a great friendship.

Over the next few months, we were completely inseparable. We grew closer and closer and started to fall in love.

I still had a tremendous amount of weight to lose, and he felt he needed to drop a few pounds, so we started a weight loss program together. We did it faithfully, every day, until the end of the program. With his support, I lost almost all of the weight I had gained over the last four years.

The most amazing thing about him, though, was that my weight did not matter. All he cared about was keeping me healthy.

We talked many times about CFIDS and how it affected me. My parents explained to him how CFIDS had impacted their life. We tried to impress on him how dramatically CFIDS changed all of us.

But there was nothing to worry about, we thought. After all, getting better quality sleep seemed to solve any problems I'd had before.

This was my healthiest time ever. I was sleeping well and feeling great. I worked out everyday and my diet was good. I think Mike believed CFIDS was part of my history and not my future.

There was no way to prepare him for what was to come.

In September 2001, seven months after we met, I went to Dr. Jones for my routine Pap smear. During the breast exam, she commented that she felt something strange, and I should follow up on it. I had a mammogram and ultrasound that day. The radiologist agreed with Dr. Jones and recommended seeing a surgeon.

During this same time, I started having minor speech problems. I was tripping over my tongue, and found it difficult to say words I was thinking. I also noticed my joints were hurting, but in the past few months, had dismissed it and figured I had worked out too hard.

I began noticing problems with my sight. Mike and I were driving one day and, all of a sudden, I lost the peripheral vision in my right eye. We immediately went to the emergency room, and after a six-hour wait, found out I'd had an eye migraine. This sounded valid; I had suffered from migraines for ten years, and after we left the emergency room, I did not think much of it.

Finally, I was experiencing bad heart palpitations. My blood pressure was very low and my heart rate was extremely high. My heart skipped beats, and would feel like it was going to pound out of my chest when I was lying down.

I started by going to the surgeon for the lump in my breast. He believed it was a benign fibrocystic mass — clumps of fatty tissue — and did not feel a biopsy was necessary, but understood if I wanted one. I was still extremely scared, and because of all of the problems I was having felt it would not hurt to have the biopsy done. It was scheduled for the next week.

Then I went to Dr. Smith. He ran a test to check for Lupus because of the joint pain, scheduled a cardiac ultrasound, and decided to do a MRI for multiple sclerosis.

The cardiac ultrasound showed a mild mitral valve prolapse on one side of the heart. It can cause the valve to not close completely. Fortunately, the finding is not uncommon and he decided to keep an eye on it and not pursue treatment at that time. My test for Lupus came back irregular, and I was referred to a rheumatologist.

I sat down with the rheumatologist, and he reviewed my test results. I explained to him that over the last few months, I had gone off the birth control pill and quit the anti-depressant I had been on and told him that I was hoping to avoid using any medication. I felt I was doing better without the chemicals.

He set the papers down, looked me square in the eyes and said, "Then why are you here?"

Horrified, I answered, "To find out if I have Lupus."

"But what does it matter if you're not willing to be chemically treated?" he quipped.

"I'll consider treatment if you can tell me whether or not I have Lupus!" I said, frustrated.

After a cursory exam, he decided I did not have Lupus and quickly sent me on my way.

The MRI was going to be quite expensive, and I decided to go to my primary care physician to see if he would order the test so that my out of pocket expense would be less. I scheduled an appointment and Mike and I went to the office.

We signed in and sat down. Within a few minutes I was called into the exam room.

We only waited a short time for the doctor to come in. He opened the door, walked over to the counter, opened the chart, and looked at me.

"What can I do for you?" he asked.

I started explaining that I have CFIDS, and he stopped me, mid-sentence.

"Are you sure you're not depressed?" He sounded annoyed.

"I'm not depressed." I was trying his patience.

"Why?" the doctor asked almost rolling his eyes.

"I'm not depressed, I'm sick," I said discouraged — and angry.

He was another doctor added to the long list of those who did not believe CFIDS patients.

He bristled and explained, in all his medical glory that, "Chronic Fatigue Syndrome doesn't exist, it's a manifestation of depression, if you get the depression controlled, you'll be fine."

He immediately left and returned a few moments later with a referral to a rheumatologist.

"I don't think this doctor will be able to help you, but if you don't want to believe you're depressed, you can try," the doctor said.

I could see the anger in Mike's face, and he could not keep quiet anymore.

"How can you say that CFIDS doesn't exist when millions of people suffer from it?" Mike questioned.

"As I told you, it's a manifestation of depression," the doctor balked.

Mike stood up, reached out to shake his hand and said, "I'm sorry we've wasted your precious time."

When the doctor reached his hand out, Mike grabbed it firmly and did not let it go. There was a very slight spark of fear in the doctor's eyes. After a moment, Mike released his grip and the doctor stepped back.

"You didn't waste my time," the doctor replied defensively.

Mike chuckled, "You walked in here, haven't laid a finger on her, and tell her that she's making up her symptoms."

The doctor was visibly shaken and started to raise his voice, "Hey, I spent five minutes talking to her, and I think she's depressed."

"Okay, fine," Mike said, looking at me, "let's go. We're obviously wasting our time!"

I did everything I could not to cry until we got in the elevator. I fought the tears and screamed at my body and mind to keep control.

Do not give this jerk the satisfaction of seeing me cry.

We finally made it to the elevator and when the doors closed, I sobbed.

"This is what I have been through for the past fifteen years; it's the same story over and over again!"

Mike was so angry he could hardly speak. I think for the first time, he understood why I felt so betrayed by the medical community.

I decided to have my MRI done through my insurance and pay whatever I had to pay. After all, it was worth any amount of money to not be treated like that again.

I scheduled my MRI for the day before my breast biopsy.

I have never been claustrophobic, and I was not worried about the MRI. I was far more concerned about the possible results. I wanted a diagnosis other than CFIDS so bad, but multiple sclerosis was not a good diagnosis to have.

I walked into the room that housed the MRI machine and kept telling myself I was fine. I got on the table and put my head in the trough.

I was a little concerned and I felt my heart rate start to rise as the technician put huge foam pads on either side of my head. She then strung tape across my forehead that was attached, on either side, to the table. Finally, she put something like a mock football helmet over my face, and started to move me back into the machine.

I started to panic slightly — my head was strapped down and I could not move it. Halfway in the tube, I got control of myself and took some deep breaths to calm down. *This is crazy!* My mind screamed. *Get control of yourself!*

Once I relaxed, the MRI was no problem. Fortunately, I found out a few days later, the scan was negative.

The biopsy ended up being a lot easier than I thought. The hardest part was the anticipation. I was so scared, but the nurse and the surgeon were both very kind. The nurse held my hand while the doctor injected an anesthetic into me.

I felt a very tiny stick and then nothing but some slight pressure. He took quite a few samples, and he kept me distracted by talking about animals. It was over in about ten minutes.

I left the office and was sore for the next day or two. The office called the next Monday with my results. The mass was benign, just some fibrocystic tissue.

Through all of these problems, Mike stood by my side. But the stress caused me to relapse within a month and I was back in bed.

I could not stay at his condominium while I was sick because there was major construction on his building and I was not able sleep.

He could not come to my house because I had two cats and he was so allergic that he had not spent more than ten minutes inside my house at any given time.

So unfortunately, our time together was limited to about once a week for a few hours.

Mike and I were struggling. Our relationship was fragile. He refused to allow me to tell him to deal with it, and for the first time, someone was holding me responsible for my actions.

I loved him more than I could explain, but I was so sick I could not address his needs. We would argue constantly about my indifference while I was sick and he struggled to understand how I felt.

He looked for some way to grasp what was happening to the person he loved. He said he was more than prepared for the physical aspect of the disease through the conversations we'd had when I was well, but he was not at all ready for the emotional turmoil.

He was mad and jealous of the disease for taking me away from him. He went through a phase where he thought I was using it as an excuse to see other people.

He could not understand that I was fighting for my life. I did not have the energy to help him through this. I begged him to get professional help or find a friend he could talk to.

Everything he had known was being yanked out from under him. His best friend was gone. I was a shell of what he knew.

I wanted him to understand that he needed to keep living. Just because I was sick did not mean he had to stay in bed too.

It took awhile, but he soon started to accept the new reality. He started to spend time with friends and make plans without me. I was always invited, but he understood if I did not make it.

He started to drop in and check on me while I was asleep. Even though he could only stay a few minutes at a time, it made him feel better to know I was all right.

When I first got sick, he really thought I might die from the disease, and was afraid he might come over and find me dead in my bed. He figured that, at least if I stayed at his house, he would know I was safe. But that, unfortunately, was not an option at the time.

It soon became easier though. I decided to stop fighting so hard and I tried to remember this was someone I loved, and someone I wanted to keep in my life.

I learned I had better get control of myself and started to treat him like my partner and friend. It was hard for me to accept and admit I was being selfish. I struggled so hard to exist each day, but all he wanted was a small sign I still cared. An occasional kind word, a loving gesture, and the feeling I loved him was all he asked for.

In the past, I became hollow when I was sick. I "holed-up" and did not want to speak to or deal with anyone. But that was not fair to do to someone I claimed to love. I worked hard to maintain my existence and still keep my best friend.

After six months, I slowly started to feel better. Mike and I knew we had made it through the eye of the storm. We were able to go out once in awhile and do the things a couple does.

We went to dinner, saw movies, and spent time with friends. It was a slow recovery, but our relationship was stronger than ever.

We knew that the next time, if there were a next time, we would be able to handle it better. After all of the pain we had experienced, we knew we were meant to be.

Mike proposed, and we set a date to get married. Despite my health problems, he still loved me, and was willing to help me through it.

He has made me a better person and given me hope. I see now that I can be loved and I look forward to having children with him. We truly are best friends. I cannot imagine life without him.

I look forward to my upcoming marriage to him, and the wonderful life we have started to share. He has been a driving force in my life. He has forever changed the way I see the world.

We do not have a perfect relationship, but we have made it through more pain and anguish than most people experience in their entire lives. We have been able to figure out a way that works for us, crazy as those ways are sometimes. And best thing of all, we just "get" each other.

We live as though CFIDS does not exist in our lives, but I

think it always lingers in the back of our heads. Knowing I might become ill again is a reality that strikes fear in both our hearts. But we try to live each day without concern for what CFIDS has in store for us.

We are planning our wedding and have booked a wonderful honeymoon with no regard for what CFIDS is doing during that time. We have plans to try to get pregnant and look forward to our future.

And best of all, Mike has taught me to live my life without consulting CFIDS. I do not care what it thinks and the threat of another attack is no longer going to run my life!

Whoever said there is no such thing as a knight in shining armor never had the pleasure of meeting Mike.

Closing

$\mathcal{I}$ have learned so much over the years, and have grown in so many ways. I used to fight every aspect of this disease, and I would not accept or even admit I was sick.

I would drag myself around on the verge of collapse before I would admit I needed help, and I refused give in to the fact that I could not work anymore. I have finally acknowledged the possibility that the constant mental fighting has contributed to my declining health over the years.

I guess, after being in bed for months at a time, maybe I finally stopped fighting just long enough to allow myself to heal. Then, when I was back on my feet, I started the fight all over again. Slowly, the same war wore me down until I could no longer fight anymore, and the cycle continued.

The hardest lesson for me to learn has been acceptance. I used to believe acceptance was synonymous with giving up, but it is not.

I no longer search tirelessly for the silver bullet, and I have stopped fighting with the CFIDS diagnosis. I do not get my hopes up every time I read an article about a cure or see an advertisement with a quick fix. Why should I be repeatedly devastated when the dream does not become a reality? I am done running from doctor to doctor, and trying drug after drug after drug.

I still remain aware of the new treatments and research and I try to stay informed about my disease. I truly believe where there is knowledge, there lies power.

If there is a next time, and I find myself in bed again, I will strive to accept it.

It is time for me to be all right with my given path.

I am tired of fighting so hard!

I have learned no matter what happens — or how sick I become, I am still a good person. I know now I have something to give and share with others. I have created meaning in my life, and I have learned to hold tight to those things I love and cherish.

At last I have been able to place some value on my life. That has been Mike's amazing contribution.

I still live my life knowing CFIDS is always lurking in the background — waiting to pounce. It hopes I become weak from the stresses of every day so it can attack and sink its teeth in.

But even with this knowledge, I continue to live my life.

I am learning to refrain from pushing too hard, and now do everything in my power to stop emotionally sabotaging myself with self-doubt and insecurity.

I do not beat myself up anymore if I feel like going to sleep at seven in the evening. I have learned not to criticize myself for sleeping nine or ten hours at night. I accept it as part of who I am. And I have given up trying to make excuses.

I no longer feel the need to justify myself to anyone. It is okay for me to say that I am tired and it is all right if I do not feel well enough to go out.

I do not work so hard trying to make everyone else happy and comfortable with my illness by justifying, making excuses, and minimizing my pain. It is what it is. Through education I hope the public can learn to make patients comfortable with their diagnosis — instead of the other way around.

I have stopped listening to the tremendous amount of criticism and realized ignorance breeds fear. Those who cannot understand CFIDS find it easiest to shove it — and its victims — in a corner and ignore them.

My internal battle is quieting, and my soul and spirit are winning more often. Over the last year, hope has replaced hopelessness, health has replaced illness, happiness has replaced fear, and acceptance has replaced complete despair.

I know that if I never become sick again, my life has been forever altered by CFIDS. I pride myself now in my strength of character as well as my patience, and compassion. Before, I consumed myself with fear, shame, guilt, and self-doubt, but all of those feelings are starting to fade into my past.

Writing this book not only helped me reflect on my struggle but also allowed me to be truthful with myself for the first time. I was able to identify the pain and anguish I felt daily — and in a way I never thought possible.

I hope those reading my story can relate to the powerful struggle I have been through and find some way to accept their own plight. For it is acceptance that gets me through each day.

Acceptance has allowed my mind to find peace — something I never knew until recently. The peace to accept life with this disease, the peace to be able to quiet my mind at night, and the peace to be happy with who I am (even though I am not the same as I was).

I have learned to love my new self, and have been able to mourn the loss of my old life. I have given up a wonderful and promising career in the animal field — knowing it played a role — and felt the huge void from that loss start to fill.

I work every day to stay positive, and I nurture myself by listening to my body. I am healthy right now, and have been for about six months. I have done everything possible to promote my emotional wellbeing and health. Even if CFIDS strikes again, a positive attitude and my emotional stability will help me get through.

My goal is to remain on that path.

It is not always easy — and sometimes I feel my internal voices try to start the battle all over again. But I am learning how to quiet them, and make them stop before they start an all-out war.

In the past, no one ever won. All there was were losers.

So now I wonder, many times, if and when CFIDS will come back. I try to stay positive and hope a pregnancy will not only help the endometriosis, but also alleviate and diminish CFIDS.

Unfortunately, only time will tell.

So I do everything in my power to spend precious little time worrying.

Instead of sitting around scared to death waiting for the next blow — I chose to get married, plan a family, and move on with my life.

I know CFIDS always remains close, but I have fought four devastating rounds with it already and am determined to learn how to abolish it from my life for good. I know I can — and I will do it!

Every day, now, I say a small thank you for being able to get out of bed, and I appreciate the love and support from Mike, my family, and the few close friends I have.

At thirty, I still have my entire life ahead of me. CFIDS or not.

And whether it is in sickness or health, I look forward to every day.

E-mail Me

I am always interested in other people's stories, both positive and negative. I believe by sharing our experiences, others can learn to cope with their own pain. Sometimes it's just nice to know you are not alone.

My goal is to continue writing my story — as it happens. For example:

- pregnancy and CFIDS
- raising children with CFIDS
- marriage and CFIDS
- people who love victims of CFIDS

Please feel free to e-mail me at:
steph@ifyouwouldjust.com

Also visit our website at **www.ifyouwouldjust.com** where you can get the latest links on CFIDS news and participate in discussion groups.